D0761441

A Difficult Journey

A DIFFICULT JOURNEY

My Battle with Cancer

Mayte Prida

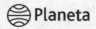
Planeta

© Mayte Prida, 2003

© Planeta Publishing Corp., 2005
  2057 NW 87 Ave.
  Miami, FL 33172 (USA)

ISBN-13: 978-1-933169-03-3
ISBN-10: 1-933169-03-6

First Edition, March 2005
Second Edition, February 2007

Photography: Carolina Attel
Printed by Printer Colombiana S. A.
Printed in Colombia

To my children, Tommy and Izzy, because with their love, support, strength and courage I have been able to face this journey.

To my parents, brothers and sister, who demonstrated their love to me.

To Papá Grande, who has been the source of inspiration and strength my whole life.

To my grandmother, who worried a lot.

To my Majito Lindo, Sandra and Juan.

INDEX

ACKNOWLEDGEMENTS

Living through a difficult journey makes us appreciate life in a different way. Not only our daily chores become different, but also the way in which we see and feel the people around us who become more special. I want to thank everybody who shared with me this arduous time, especially those who took upon themselves the responsibility of sharing their time, not only with me but, even more importantly, with my children. Their love, support and commitment made our lives a little easier during such a difficult time. I consider myself very fortunate because the list of these people is quite long. Each of them has a special place in my heart and I include them in this book as a tribute. In order to make it simpler, they are listed in alphabetical order.

Thank you,
I love you all.

Adela, for your care.
Aída, for being an inspiration in my life.
Aleksa, for coming to this world next to me.
Andrew, because you were always there.
Antonio, for being my parallel soul.
Benno, for all those magazines.
Boni, for being there along the way.
Carlos, for the belief in our mission.
Caroline, for your friendship.
Cristina, for your love and prayers.
Cristo, for your e-mails.

Doña Enriqueta, for giving me the courage to face my battle.

Doctor D., for teaching me the meaning of generosity and compassion.

Eduar, for opening up to me.

Federico, because you taught me what is real.

Felicia, for your help.

Frankie, for your massages and your friendship.

Gigi, for cheering me up.

Greg, for caring for and protecting the three of us.

Isabel, for your paellas and long talks.

Jackie, for your support.

James, for being there.

Jorge, for helping me find a meaning to my journey.

Juan, for the time you spent with me.

Juan Pablo, for the Reiki sessions.

Lilia, for your positive energy.

Manolo, for showing me that I could enjoy life again.

María, for cheering up my Tommy.

Mariló, for your friendship and support.

Mario, for protecting my business affairs.

Marquito, for your constant phone calls.

Mieke, for being my spiritual sister.

Monika, for keeping me busy on the Internet.

Monique, for your prayers and enthusiasm.

Pastor Santana and Graciela, for taking care of my children.

Phil, for teaching me how faith and medicine can walk hand in hand.

Raouf, for staying by my side.

Raúl, for motivating my children.

Rey, for your unconditional love.

Richard, for your visits and advice.

Rocío, for your constant calls.

Sandra, for sharing the whole ordeal with me.

Tere, for your true love.

Tito, for guiding my path.

Tío Chacho, for taking care of my children's tuition.

FOREWORD

Mayte Prida is a force of nature. In person, on television, and in this book, her energy, her humanity and her love of life are contagious.

My Difficult Journey, describing her battle against cancer, is a great story of personal triumph. But *My Difficult Journey* is more than the story of one brave woman's fight; it is full of wonderful insights we all can use when facing our worst fears – whether a disease or personal crisis. Importantly, Mayte hasn't just told her story and retired. In cities and towns across America, Mayte is there helping people understand more about cancer, ways to fight it, and where they can go to find help to beat it.

That is why the Pharmaceutical Research and Manufacturers of America is proud to have Mayte Prida as a spokesperson for our Partnership for Prescription Assistance (PPA) team while also leading our Hispanic outreach efforts. Her passion and eloquence in reaching across language and cultural barriers to assist Hispanic Americans with getting their medicines, inspires all who know her.

The Partnership for Prescription Assistance – sponsored by America's pharmaceutical research companies and with a big assist from Mayte – has helped nearly 4 million Americans who can't afford their prescription drugs get the medicines they need. *My Difficult Journey* reminds us all that diseases like cancer can be beaten. And Mayte Prida – in everything she does – reminds us all how important a helping hand can be.

Billy Tauzin
President and Chief Executive Officer
PhRMA

PROLOGUE

Life is beautiful, indeed. It is made up of a chain of moments created by our own experiences as we write the history of our lives in our own book. Each individual story has been written by different stages of life: happy stages, peaceful stages, tranquil stages, sad stages and difficult stages. Each one of them plays a very important role in the school of learning, through which the soul evolves.

God, who is very wise, gave me the opportunity to live very intense moments by the side of a very special human being: a brave woman who taught me and became my Master as to how to face a very painful illness that unfortunately feeds the fear in us. Cancer is basically fear and suppressed anger compressed into sad capsules.

Mayte, the author of this book, is the teacher that was able to overcome this *Difficult Journey*, which was only a stage in her beautiful and successful life. She was able to overcome it with the help of love, willingness and excitement for life—always with dignity.

One of the main lessons I learned from this great woman was that the love for life and the responsibility of taking care of two precious souls make it possible to transform a person like herself into the maker of her own miracles. I'm going to open my heart to tell you about this enriching experience.

It was a Sunday afternoon in Miami and I had been invited to a luncheon in the house of our friend, Aída. I arrived early. As soon as I walked into the living room, my eyes came in contact with the tender look of a young and beautiful woman who seemed a little tired. She was introduced to me as Mayte. We started to talk right away because we are both from Mexico and that's how we began our conversation. A special feeling blossomed that led to a very special friendship.

She told me she had just gotten out of the hospital and that it was her first time out of the house. When I asked her what was wrong with her, she told me she had cancer. I really didn't know what to say. I held her hand. Right then and there I felt that this meeting presented a very special lesson for me. At that very moment I decided that I needed to give her my emotional support and, especially, I felt that I needed to be by her side. Mother Teresa used to tell me that the most important kind of help that you can give another human being is to share with them our time, because time is the most difficult thing for human beings to share. With Mayte I wanted to share conscious moments of my time. I was with Mayte during almost all of her chemotherapies. I lived by her side during her Difficult Journey. I witnessed the tests of determination and the acceptance of her reality. Each and every day that I spent with her I admired her more because she wouldn't give up. On the contrary, she took her unpleasant and painful experience as a lesson that she needed to face on her way to becoming a better person.

In the middle of her journey she wouldn't complain. She would always observe, accept and learn. Her greatest wish was to be healthy again, to prove to her children and to herself that she was capable of fighting. I was moved by her positive attitude of wanting to give her testimony of pain and strength to others who face cancer. From the very beginning she thought that somehow she could serve as an example by facing her reality, carrying her own cross without being the victim.

During her chemotherapies we would meditate so that her body would start healing itself. We believe that the mind plays a very important role in the healing process. We were connecting her faith in God with the good of the universe. She began accepting herself, loving herself, forgiving herself, and wishing for life while caressing her soul.

One day she became very ill due to the side effects of the chemotherapies. I was by myself waiting for her at her hospital room when they wheeled her in on the stretcher. Upon seeing her I became very sad. She was very pale, scared and very cold. She was in a lot of pain because her body was not responding to the treatments. Even though she was feeling all of this, she was totally conscious, because the pain awakens the conscious and the conscious then becomes clear and receptive. We held each other. She was lying down in the stretcher as we both cried in silence. It was a meeting of our old souls reuniting again. It was a very spiritual moment. When the nurses put her into her bed she asked me to guide her in a meditation and do some praying. With her childish smile, she asked me to pray to her angels, so I began doing it. As soon as we started praying and meditating, Mayte began to reach a state of peace that almost seemed out of this world. We could feel the love that floated in the room. All I could do was utter sentences thanking God for everything that we were experiencing. Mayte was very grateful to me for helping her reach her soul and initiating her peaceful connection to God. We lost track of time because we embraced the time of the universe. It protected us and a humble miracle began to happen. Mayte's body began to respond. It was only then that the intestinal occlusion which had been one of the main problems began reversing itself. She had been in the intensive care unit for almost two days and her body had not responded to the treatments. But when Mayte's body harmonized itself with God and the universe, her body felt it and reacted.

In that way the chemo treatments progressed and, with each one of them, Mayte's soul was purifying itself through suffering. She had lost her hair and gained some weight, but believe me when I tell you that each day she looked more beautiful as she fought harder to overcome cancer.

Among the many things that I learned in this journey was that each moment in life is special and it's never the same again. Life does not stop. It is always in constant change. The word "always" doesn't exist because life moves constantly. We have to learn to let go. I believe that the hardest lesson that we have to learn on this planet earth is the art of letting go. Sooner or later all of us are going to leave this planet, but when that happens, it is only our souls that leave. Everything that we accumulate in life stays here, because to reunite with the spirit of the universe we only need our spirit, not our possessions.

Thank you, Mayte for everything I learned by your side. Through your pain and suffering I learned and grew up as a woman, a mother, a friend and a writer. Thank you for giving me such a great example. God bless you.

— LILIA REYES SPINDOLA

Note: Mrs. Reyes Spindola is one of the most recognized Mexican authors. Her work in which she writes about Angels have enriched the souls of millions.

INTRODUCTION

It is difficult to explain how the word cancer can change your life in such a radical way. Before I knew that I could die because the cancer was growing inside my body, I lived a happy and busy life. I had been living in Miami for two years at the time, during which I had grown a lot both emotionally and spiritually. The woman who had arrived with two small children was blossoming and starting to get out of her shell to experience a new world and a new reality. On those days my reality was about work, great expectations, and the conquest of new horizons. It was also about beating difficulties and a constant search to achieve new goals that helped my identity as a woman to become stronger each day. In my reality at that time, words had a different meaning than they have today. I wasn't afraid of obstacles. I didn't know the meaning of being afraid. Determination ruled my everyday life. In a way, I guess it was during this period of time, when I was about 30 years old, that I stopped being a girl and was becoming a fully mature woman.

Then my reality changed all of a sudden. I accepted and understood that I had cancer, knowing from that moment on that I was starting to live a different life. Before cancer, I worked hard to create a stable future for my children. After cancer, I was fighting simply to be able to *live* for my children. The priorities that I had before knowing that I had cancer stopped being on top of my list. From that moment on my whole life changed completely.

One of the first things I did when I knew I had this illness was to seek information. I obtained books and flyers that explained breast cancer. I downloaded pages and pages from the Internet and read about hundreds of cases similar to mine. I went to a lot of bookstores trying to find an answer and a ray of hope. Even though I had heard the word *cancer* throughout my life, I always felt that it was far removed from my family and me.

It wasn't difficult to find information about breast cancer because it has one of the highest mortality rates among women in this country. What became a challenge was to learn to disseminate all the information I had. The more scientific it got, the more statistics I found and the more scared I became. It was frightening to me to read about life span averages, the number of deaths, the number of people who recuperate, and the number of those who get it again. I didn't want to become just one more number. I was very confused. I didn't know how to start facing my new reality.

That's how one day, feeling lost in the middle of all this information, I started feeling a reason to find a meaning for my situation. That's when I thought that maybe my own experience could serve as a guide, inspiration, hope or comfort to somebody else who would suddenly face a problem similar to mine.

I do not like to play the role of a victim. I have never done it and I wasn't about to start, but my personal situation at the time of being diagnosed with cancer was extremely difficult. If I was to write a classified ad for a newspaper, I would describe it like this: Divorced woman, single mother with two financially dependant children, without a stable job nor a fixed salary, living off her savings, with a huge debt, fighting in court with ex-husband, living in a strange country in a city without relatives, and living without medical insurance in a society in which doctors make more money than educators or politicians. Woman, dreamer, idealist, optimist and a fighter.

I am one of those who preach that in life we shouldn't compare because I believe that we are all different and need to accept each other the way we are. Everyone's realities are individual and very different because our own beliefs and experiences influence these realities. I know that there are many women suffering from breast cancer just like me whose situations might be much more difficult than mine and that they have made it. But I also know that there are women that have a much better prognosis than mine but, for one reason or another, don't make it.

In this book I write about my own particular case, my personal situation and the way in which I was facing obstacles and blessings along the way. I write about my life and the way in which I had to face my situation. My attitude was pretty firm from the moment I understood my new reality. Once the problem was diagnosed I needed to find the solution.

Since I was little girl, I have been writing diaries. Every now and then I enjoy reading them just to see how my life has passed, so it was easy for me to be documenting the stages I was going through. At the same time, taking advantage of the technical equipment in my office, I documented on video, step by step, my new reality, especially during the most relevant days. One day I gave each one of my children a notebook. We decorated the covers, writing "My Cancer Book" on each of them. I asked them to write about their feelings and emotions whenever they felt the need to do so. I did this initially as a form of therapy for them. But now I include some of their writings in my book because what my children felt and lived during my Difficult Journey is also felt and lived by thousands of children around the world every single day of the year.

When my problem was diagnosed, we didn't know what kind of ending it would have. Even today we do not know the end of this chapter of my life because cancer is a very vicious illness, the results of which are measured by statistics. I do not agree with that. I want to somehow contribute to help spread the understanding of how difficult life can be, not only for those of us who suffer from the illness, but also for our families, our friends, and those who love us and are with us during this time. I want to prove that there is always a ray of light and hope along the way no matter how dark a situation may be.

With this illness I have learned a lot. I have discovered new facets of life that were unknown to me. I have understood what faith is, what friendship is, and what unconditional love is, and what compassion, help, support and hope truly are. I have come across the goodness of people. I have discovered that love is what really moves the world. I have been very happily surprised. Although I was deceived by a couple of selfish people, I chose to see the good rather than the bad in every situation, having learned even from them.

Throughout my life I have had the opportunity of being a leader. I don't care how small a leader is, a leader always has followers. As I said before, my personal situation at the time of finding the cancer was extremely difficult in many aspects. But with the help of God Father and Mother, the Supreme Being, the Universe, the Guardian Angels, my Protectors and my Spiritual Guides, my spiritual family, my family, my friends, and the kindness and generosity of so many people, even total strangers, I have been able to make it.

That is why, as a testimony of this year—the most difficult of my life—I want to express in writing this book the experiences that I've had in gratitude to the universe for having given me the opportunity of finding so much love, care, compassion and generosity around me. Even though this has really been a very Difficult Journey, it has also been the period of time in which I have received a lot of blessings, opportunities for growth and personal satisfaction. This is a year for which I will be eternally grateful.

Cancer does not discriminate. It is a bad and treacherous illness. It doesn't play a fair game. It hides in the most inner places of our bodies and starts growing for months, making us sick without even a warning. It is a coward. It doesn't have a face. It is bad and one day, if we do not find out about its existence, it simply steals our life away.

I am a woman. I am a mother. I am a friend. And I want to share with you some of my experiences with the purpose of delivering a ray of hope in the middle of the darkness, isolation, doubt, fear and imbalance that is created by cancer. If I am able to inspire or motivate one life, I will be satisfied that I had returned to the universe some of the knowledge that I received during this very Difficult Journey.

DISCOVERING THE TUMOR

It was six in the morning on the second Sunday of February. As I was stepping out of the shower, I realized that my towel wasn't hanging in its usual place. Dripping with water, I made an unusual gesture with my arm trying to reach for another towel from its hanger. At a glance, I was able to see my breasts in the bathroom mirror and noticed something that looked like a good size lump on the lower part of my right breast. Hoping that it was just a shadow, I lowered my arms, dried myself off and looked in the mirror. I didn't see a thing. I raised my arm again in the same way in which I had it when I was trying to reach for the towel and I saw the lump again. "No! Please!" I told myself. I got very close to the mirror and felt a real hard lump. Looking at it, it seemed like a marble inside my skin. I was afraid. I stepped out of the bathroom and sat at the edge of my bed, thinking of what I should do and asking myself which doctor I should call. At that time I realized that it was Sunday, that I was ready to go shoot the last segments of our new pilots for the season, and that there was nothing I could do until Monday. I tried not to give it a lot of importance. I got dressed and left my house.

On my way to the location of the pilot shoot, I touched my breast each time that I was stopped at a traffic signal, trying to double check if the lump was real. I knew that it was there, but I was so afraid that I wanted to think I had imagined it.

When I got to the location, I met with Antonio, my great friend and coworker, and I mentioned to him what I had found. I explained to him that I was really afraid. He was a little bit doubtful and tried not to give much importance to the problem, telling me that more than likely it was just a cyst. Nevertheless, he made it very clear that I needed to call the doctor early the next morning. For the first time in years, the hours of shooting seemed like an eternity. Besides the anxiety that I was beginning to feel when I thought about the lump, the work ambiance that day was particularly tense for other reasons.

First thing on Monday I phoned my gynecologist's office trying to make an appointment to see him. As usually, no one answered the phone, so I left a message on their answering machine and went to my office. Three hours later I hadn't heard from the doctor or the nurse. I tried phoning again with no luck. Two hours later, now in a bad mood and a little nervous, I called one more time determined not to hang up the phone until the receptionist actually answered. Once she did, I told her that I needed to speak to the doctor and that, if she didn't let me talk to him, I was going to go sit outside his reception area until he could see me. That was the only way she would give me an appointment in between scheduled patients for the following day.

I arrived at to the doctor's office and sat in the waiting area for about an hour and a half. I had met this doctor when I had just moved to Miami because I had some pre-cancerous issues in the past. That's why I was very careful to do routine checkups every six months. Once inside the examining room, he checked me, feeling the lump. He told me that it didn't look good. He said I definitely needed to investigate what it was and ordered a mammogram and an ultrasound. I was very worried, especially after he told me I needed to wait at least five days before having the exams due to fact that it was the first day of my menstrual cycle, which could give false results.

I went home a little bit frustrated but I wasn't that worried because the doctor seemed relaxed. As soon as I got home, I called Antonio to tell him what the doctor had said and he suggested that we call his brother-in-law, Tito, a pathologist in Miami. He thought it would be a good idea to tell him about my findings just to get some medical advice. I doubted it a little bit because I didn't feel that I had enough confidence to call him, even though I had met him socially on a few occasions, so Antonio called him on my behalf. One of the greatest blessings along my process began at that very moment.

I called the hospital to try to make an appointment for the exams the following week, but they told me that the first available date was three weeks later. I couldn't believe it. I was disappointed for having had to wait for such a long time. I decided to call Tito myself to ask him if he could call the hospital where he worked to arrange an appointment so that I could get the exams sooner. He was able to get me into the hospital a week later. It was a Monday holiday and my friend and coworker, Juan, had offered to go with me so I wouldn't have to go by myself. He waited for me outside. I had the mammogram done and then they took me to a room where the nurse started to perform an ultrasound. I tried to make conversation with her, but she was very quiet with me. I know now that for legal reasons, the hospital doesn't allow technicians to communicate with patients. At that time, however, I thought she just didn't want to talk to me and, assuming she didn't want to say something that would compromise her job. After performing the sonogram for some time, she stepped out of the room. A while later she came back with the doctor whom Tito had said would be examining me. They both proceeded to examine my right breast again. The doctor simply looked at me, saying that she was going to send the results of my exam to my gynecologist and to Tito. She told me that they would be the ones in charge of giving me the final diagnosis. Before stepping out of the room she told me that it didn't look good, that there was definitely a big tumor, and that I needed to start looking for a surgeon to remove it. She paused for a second. Looking straight at me, she asked if I knew of any oncologists.

I pretended to be very brave, but I just felt my world collapsing. "An oncologist?" I asked myself. I went to the dressing room and put on my clothes again. I wanted to cry so badly, but tried not to because I had to go to the cashier to pay and I didn't want everyone to see how worried I was. Right outside the door was Juan, who knew by just looking at me that something was wrong. He held my hand and didn't say a word, waiting to ask me what had happened until we got into the car. I couldn't talk. I simply started to cry. I was crying and crying. Between sobs, I told him that I thought it was cancer because the doctor had asked me if I knew an oncologist. I couldn't stop crying and I was asking out loud: "What's going to happen to my children? What's going to happen to my children? What's going to happen to them?" Even though I didn't have the official results of the test, the way the doctor and the nurse reacted and the advice to get an oncologist had made it pretty clear that I had cancer. I just knew it.

A couple of hours later, my gynecologist called me to tell me that the lump was a malignant tumor. He gave me the names and phone numbers of two medical oncologists for me to call. By the tone of his voice, I could tell that he was sorry about my situation. He told me that his participation as a doctor was ending right there, but he wanted me to keep him informed of the progress.

I called the oncologist's office to try to make an appointment and they told me that the doctor was not available until the end of March. I asked, "The end of March? This is only the middle of February! I have a tumor inside, they told me it is bad, and I don't know exactly what it is, and you are asking me to wait six weeks before meeting the doctor?" Very frustrated, mad and nervous, I hung up the phone and simply started to cry.

After crying for a while I decided that I needed some more help, so I called Tito again and asked him for guidance. He knew of the results and happened to be a very good friend of the oncologist. He asked me to relax and take it easy, adding that he would call him personally to ask him to see me without having to wait for such a long time. He did it. Four days later, I met for the first time with Doctor D., my surgeon oncologist and another one of my Angels along the way.

THE DIAGNOSIS

"The first day that my mommy had cancer, I felt very, very bad. I was afraid and very worried because I thought she was going to die. I wanted to believe that she was going to be all right, but I was very afraid. When she started going to the doctors and the hospital, my little sister, Izzy, cried a lot. She was also very afraid, but I kept telling her not to cry anymore because mommy was going to be all right. I was very worried to see my little sister sooooo sad."

— Tommy

After waiting anxiously for four days, the time to meet with Doctor D., the oncologist, finally arrived. It was a Friday afternoon. Antonio had offered to go with me and I agreed because I didn't want to go by myself. I was afraid of the confirmation of the bad news.

Besides being totally afraid of the illness, I was worried about what cancer would mean for me financially without medical insurance. I had no idea what was going to happen in that meeting. I didn't know how long I was going to be there and I didn't even know if they were going to do a biopsy. I had asked Tom, my ex-husband and the father of my children, to pick them up from school and take care of them over the weekend. I had the feeling that if they were going to do a biopsy on me, I wasn't going to be in the mood to go home and do household chores. Besides that, I needed to be alone to think about what was happening to me.

After filling out the paperwork at the oncologist's office, Antonio and I sat for a while in the waiting area. I started to observe the women who were sitting near me. At least eight of them were visibly older than I am. They would not talk among themselves. They were reading a magazine or simply staring at the wall. It gave me the impression that we were all there waiting for a stiff sentence. I then understood why they had told me that I had to wait six weeks to see the doctor, because there was a constant flow of women coming in and out while I was there. I was very grateful to Tito for helping me so that the doctor would see me so soon. I knew that he had made a special concession to see me because I was Tito's friend.

After waiting a little more than an hour, the doctor's assistant took me into a room where I waited for about 10 more minutes. I could hear the doctor's voice coming from the next room. With each minute that passed I grew more nervous. He knocked on the door and came in. His physical appearance was completely different from what I had imagined. When he started talking, he had a very strong foreign accent, which I later learned was from Armenia. He introduced himself and made me feel welcome by telling me that he was really looking forward to meeting me because Tito had spoken very highly of me. Even though I was trying hard to hide my nervousness, he knew how I was feeling. Without making me wait any longer, he asked me for the X-rays and ultrasound results. He switched on the light to look at them, took out a ruler, and observed them very slowly. With a very tranquil and confident voice, he told me that he was going to do a biopsy right then and there. He explained that the biopsy was simply a routine procedure, that he had been practicing his specialty for more than 20 years, and that by looking at the X-rays and sonogram he knew I definitely had breast cancer.

For a while I didn't know what to do. The confirmation of the news was so overwhelming. I felt my nose turning red and my eyes trying to fight back the tears. He stepped out of the room for a moment, allowing me to undress and put on the hospital gown. He came back a few minutes later to proceed with the biopsy.

He performed what in medical terms is known as a fine needle aspiration biopsy, which means that the needle is stuck right into the tumor to extract the liquid from it. He did not use any anesthetic for this procedure and the truth is that it was extremely painful. Once he extracted the liquid, he transferred it into a little clear container and asked his secretary to call a messenger to take the sample to Tito, who was waiting at the hospital to analyze it.

While I was listening to all of this, I was lying on the hospital bed. I was so afraid that I thought I was going to faint. Seeing that I was turning pale, the doctor himself went to get me a glass of water and helped me to drink it. He stepped out of the room again after asking me to put my clothes back on.

After a few minutes, he came back into the room again, sat down in front of me, and told me, "There is a Chinese Proverb that says, 'The longest journey begins with the first step.' You are taking your first step today of what is going to be a long journey. Your tumor is pretty big; it is approximately 3.8 centimeters, which indicates that the cancer is in an advanced stage. I don't know exactly if it is stage two or three, or if it is still just contained in the breast, or if it has metastasized. There is a genuine possibility that it has already extended to your lymph nodes and other places, which is only going to aggravate the situation. I do not want to jump to conclusions. I want you to know that this is a delicate situation that we are going to handle in the best possible way. While we wait for the results from pathology, we need to talk about a plan of action. The first thing we need to do is to operate on you to remove the tumor and analyze where the cancer has expanded. There is no specific reason why I would think you are suffering from cancer, but you have to be brave and face it."

I couldn't contain my tears any longer. They were just rolling down my cheeks, even though I was wearing glasses. I was trying to understand my new reality, a very harsh one that was officially beginning at that precise moment. A reality that will radically change my life: I had breast cancer.

I considered myself to be a brave woman of strong character. I have been afraid many times in my life, but I never felt as terrified as I was at that moment and during many months after that. Starting that day, I learned a new meaning of the word "fear" and I had no choice but to learn to live with it. It is a fear of the unexpected and of the uncontrollable. It is a fear that is very hard to explain.

In my mind, scenes of my life quickly flashed before me as if I was watching a movie in fast motion. I couldn't believe what was happening to me. Just a month ago I was welcoming the New Year in Spain at the Virgin of Rocío Church while enjoying time with friends. At that moment my life was full of expectations. Professionally speaking, I was starting to work on what I thought was going to be a year of success. But then, I was sitting there and the doctor was telling me that I had cancer! Cancer? Me? I asked these questions a thousand times. It's not possible. It's not possible that it is happening to me. I kept thinking there must be a mistake.

Doctor D. realized my state of confusion and fear. He handed me a tissue so that I could wipe my tears. I felt his compassion and begged him to help me. I told him how fearful and confused I was and that I had two little children. I had so many doubts in my mind. Even though I wanted to know more about my illness, my mind kept wandering. The doctor told me that he was going to give me some time alone so that I could digest the news and then he exited the room. Being there all by myself, I kept trying to understand how it was possible that this was happening to me, since I was relatively young. I thought that I was a healthy and happy woman who had learned to enjoy life. I was trying to understand how or when the tumor had begun to grow. I kept asking myself how it was possible that I hadn't detected it earlier. Nothing made sense at that time. I kept thinking about my children, worrying about what their reaction would be after hearing the news. Cancer? Me? I kept asking myself … cancer? How can this happen to me if I am a good person. If all I do is try to lead a good life and take care of my children. Cancer? I am a single mother who can't even have a cold for two days or a backache without altering our daily life. How can I have something so bad, which may be incurable? Cancer? Cancer! It's not possible. I don't want to hear that word. Please God, I would think to myself, please not me, please let it be a mistake.

Bills, work, lack of medical insurance, rent, childcare, hospital, doctors … how am I going to do it? It's not possible! My anguish and incredulity lead the way to anger and fear. At last, the doctor walked into the room. I tried to cover up my anger and frustration, but he had a lot of experience and he talked softly to me again. He told me the sooner I accepted the reality, the better it would be for my own good. He urged me to seek a second opinion so that I would feel totally confident if I should decide to have him as my surgeon. Once again I felt compassion and, even though it's a little strange to say, a feeling of protection came over me simply by being next to that man. Looking back on it, I think there was a spiritual connection with him. His white hair inspired trust. Despite the chaos of the situation, I began to feel more at ease, even though I was totally afraid and confused.

I remembered that Antonio was outside waiting for me. I wanted to run to tell him what was happening to me. Doctor D., an expert in these situations, asked me if the person who was with me was close to me because he wanted to give me his final diagnosis in his office in front of someone else. He explained to me that, in difficult situations such as that one, patients tend to block part of the information received due to the impact of the news. Therefore, he would rather give the final diagnosis to the patient while in the company of a family member or a close friend. I felt great that Antonio was there with me. A little bit later the nurse brought him to the doctor's office. When he saw me, he knew right away that it wasn't good. He simply hugged me and gave me a kiss on the forehead. I started to cry.

After a few minutes the doctor came into his office and we both sat in front of him. He explained to Antonio what he had already explained to me. He urged us to start taking action. The first thing he wanted me to get were some more specialized tests to try to find out if the cancer had metastasized, which means if it had spread to other parts of the body. While he was talking my mind was wandering. I was experiencing something very strange, as if my body was sitting right there but my mind was out of my body. I would hear what the doctor was saying, but I would wander again thinking 10,000 things at the same time. My children ... surgery ... tests ... chemotherapy ... cancer. I had a million doubts and, for the first time in my life, a real fear of death. Not of dying in itself, but because I didn't want to leave my children so young.

Antonio and I left the office and walked to the car. I couldn't even say a word. My eyes were full of tears. I couldn't talk. Right next to me, Antonio—my great friend, my angel—tried to find words to console me, but I couldn't do anything else but cry, cry and cry.

While Antonio was driving, he was trying to cheer me up. But I wasn't even paying attention to what he was saying. All I was doing was trying to understand. How could I be facing this deadly illness? He, trying to make me feel better, kept telling me that everything was going to be all right, but there was absolutely no confidence in his voice. Having gone through this experience has made me understand that times like these are very difficult not only for the patient but also for those who love them. Somehow they feel the pain that we are experiencing.

Once we got home, Antonio made sure that I was feeling good enough to be alone. He had to leave because he was acting on a movie shoot. As soon as I closed the door behind him, I started crying again, only this time without holding back. I knelt down next to a wall in my bedroom, crying uncontrollably. My cry was so loud. It came from the deepest part of my soul, carrying with it the enormous pain that I was feeling.

That night I practically did not sleep because I spent the night crying. I kept turning in bed from one side to the other, but each time I moved my breast would hurt because of the biopsy I had had, reminding me of my new difficult reality. I kept crying and trying to make a mental plan of action, but confusion and fear kept returning. It was a really difficult night during which I kept asking myself many times: What's going to happen to my children? How is this going to change their lives? What are they going to think about it? What are they going to be feeling? How are they going to deal with it? The only good thing that I could think of was to be grateful that I was the one with the illness and not one of them.

The night felt like an eternity. I couldn't stop thinking about the innocence of my children and the tremendous responsibility that this would bring upon them. The three of us had been very close our whole lives. Perhaps, from a selfish point of view, I didn't want them to grow up without me. That was my main fear of death, because I am a person who believes in the evolution of life and I always have looked at death as a natural consequence to life. I have always believed that we are simply souls and our bodies are something like our wardrobes, which eventually have to be abandoned while our spirit remains alive.

All night long I kept wondering about the severity of my situation. I wanted to find answers to so many questions, such as finding the solution to come up with the money to pay for the cure and what would be the right course of action to take.

I have always believed that when we are going through a very intense stage of pain, a great loss, a sense of betrayal, it's extremely important to feel the emotions profoundly so that we can set them free. I think it is very important to feel the pain to its fullest extent, because that's the only way in which we can let go of it. I believe that once we hit rock bottom pain, reaching that place where we can go no further any longer, we have no choice but to come back from it. I believe that on that night I cried as many tears as was humanly possible. I felt the pain deep inside of my soul. I felt the fear to the fullest extent. After experiencing these feelings, I had to release them and start facing them. I didn't know what was coming, but once I understood how serious the situation was, I had no choice but to face it. As soon as the sun rose the following morning, I stared at the blue ocean on a beautiful sunny day, telling myself: "I have this huge problem, now I need to find a solution." With my eyes totally swollen after all that crying, I had a small smile on my face, because from that moment on I decided I was going to fight as hard as I could to try to live. I came up with the conclusion that cancer was another obstacle in my life, but I wasn't going to let it win the battle. At the very least, I wasn't going to let it invade my body, because from that moment on I was going to fight as hard as I could to get rid of it. I knew it was the beginning of a long battle that I was going to try to win. If I didn't win it, at least cancer was going to battle with me consciously and it was going to fight a long fight. With this new attitude, I decided to start calling my family and friends to deliver the bad news.

PHONE CALLS

The first phone call that I made to let my loved ones know about the results of my diagnosis was to my mother. It wasn't easy. A few days before, I had spoken to her by telephone to let her know they had found a tumor and that the doctor had ordered a mammogram and an ultrasound. While that conversation was taking place, I was afraid because I sensed that something was going to be wrong. Following a normal reaction, she tried to make me feel that it wasn't a big deal. This time I had the results. They were frightening. My life had changed drastically overnight.

I have never liked giving bad news, especially over the phone because I find it very impersonal. But due to the fact that the members of our family lived so far away in different countries, I had to do it like that. I was pretending to be strong, but after a little while I couldn't hold it anymore. I crumbled and started to cry. The confusion that the results created and the emotional pain were so huge that I didn't know how to resume my normal life. I told her over and over that what worried me the most was my children. I thought that being a mother herself she could understand me. I needed somebody to cheer me up to give me confidence and to give me support.

Throughout my life I have learned that people don't necessarily react the way we wish they would because everybody reacts to the same situation in the way they know best. In this particular situation, my mother started talking and talking and talking, giving me advice on how I should face the problem financially and how I needed to modify my lifestyle to make it easier on others. It's interesting, but it was the first time that I got this kind of advice, which was designed to ease somebody else's situation and not necessarily my own. I think I learned a lot about the philosophy of life by listening to her, to some of my uncles and to my brothers, all of whom advised me on the drastic changes I needed to make to my lifestyle. During all these conversations, I started to realize that it is very easy to give advice to people about how to live their lives. But the reality was that nobody was walking in my shoes and nobody really knew my situation or me. Therefore, I thought nobody had the right to impose his or her opinion.

One of the first bits of advice that my mother gave me that day was to move out of my apartment in Miami and to relocate to Mazatlan, Mexico, where she lives, so that she could keep an eye on me. She told me that for her it would be easier to help me that way because she wouldn't have to quit her job to spend time with me. Besides the fact that financially I would be better off if I was paying for all the medical treatments in Mexican pesos as opposed to U.S. dollars.

I tried to remain calm and at ease. I truly thanked her good intentions, but told her very firmly that I had no plans of changing my lifestyle. It was perfectly clear to me that after the diagnosis our stability as a family was being affected. I wanted to maintain my daily routines so that my children would feel less stressed about the situation.

I think the first conversation with my mother augmented the confusion that I was facing because her ideas and suggestions intensified my anguish, my fear, and all my feelings. I ended the phone call extremely sad, afraid and confused. After hanging up the phone, I sat down in a corner of my room and put my head between my knees, crying desperately.

I believe that as human beings we are good by nature, but that sometimes the lives we live can change or alter that very same nature. I have learned that a lot of people love giving advice, but their good advice is not necessarily what works for you. In my case in particular, a lot of my relatives told me that I needed to move out of my "expensive" apartment in Miami and that I needed to move back to Mexico. But nobody ever told me, "I'm giving you a check so you can pay for your move and come live with us." Nor did they ever tell me, "You and the children can come live with us for a period of time." Since that never happened, I simply thanked everybody for his or her advice and decided to continue living my life in the same fashion that I had been living it. To tell the truth, it was a little bit difficult for me to understand why so many people insisted in me changing my lifestyle to make it easier on them when I was the one living with the problem.

After speaking with my mother and crying in the room for a long, long time, I decided to move on with my life and started calling my friends to tell them the results of my biopsy. Some of them knew about my appointment with the doctor and had been calling and leaving messages on my answering machine, trying to find out what was going on.

The first calls I made were not easy because as soon as I said, "I have cancer," my eyes would get teary and my voice was trembling. After a few calls, I started to realize that talking about the problem kind of put it into a different perspective. After a handful of conversations, I finally started to assimilate the situation in a better way. That particular day I learned how we are all different in the way in which we react to the same situation. I faced totally different reactions from my friends. Without a doubt, all of them were worried about my condition and some couldn't believe that it could happen to me. A couple of times, I had to be the strong one because some of my friends were so worried about me that they started crying. What really sticks in my mind is the reaction of two of my good girlfriends, because they were so anguished and worried that they scared me more than I was already scared. All of a sudden, I found myself trying to convince them that everything was going to be all right. I kept telling them that I was going to fight this and wasn't about to let it win over my body. From that day on I started to realize that, no matter how similar we think we are, we all don't see life or death with the same perspective. I understood that some of us are stronger when we have to react to a certain situation. I believe that these phone calls represented the beginning of my acceptance of the problem.

Four days after receiving the diagnosis, the news about my illness was circulating rapidly among my circle of friends and acquaintances. I decided that it would be better if I delivered the news directly to them rather than have them talk about it behind my back. I'm writing about these experiences because I think it is important to understand that not everybody reacted the way I thought they would or the way I would have. When talking about my condition to some of my friends, some tried to make it seem less important than it was so that I wouldn't feel bad. They said things like, "Don't worry about it, it's not as bad as you think; I know of such and such a person and she's cured," or "It's not that bad, my aunt had the same thing and she's fine today." Some of them, in trying to make me feel good, would tell me the story of somebody they knew who fought for several years trying to win the battle; unfortunately, those people had lost the battle and knowing about that made both of us feel bad.

Trying to deal with all these disappointments is not easy. I frequently heard my friends saying things like, "Your case is not that bad," or "I've known of a lot of cases worse than yours." Although I know all those comments were made with good intentions as a way of trying to make the problem look smaller than it was, I honestly believe that sometimes it is better to let the patient feel his or her pain and deal with it in their own way without making comparisons to other people's cases. I believe that comparing similar situations is not necessarily a good thing to do because our lives are not the same and our experiences are different. Therefore, the way we handle the situation is different. By telling people something that in our opinion is going to make them feel good can perhaps cause the exact opposite effect, thereby hurting the feelings of the person we are trying to help.

In any case, making phone calls to deliver such news is never easy. But I believe that once we start to tell those who care for us about our situation, it can be very beneficial, because the circle of love begins to form around us.

TRIP TO MEXICO

It was Saturday morning and I woke up after getting very little sleep, thinking constantly about my children and grandparents. Due to the close relationship I've had with them my whole life, I was very worried about the pain that my illness was going to cause them. Since they lived in Mexico City, I decided to fly down there that same afternoon to deliver the news in person rather than over the phone. They are elderly and, unfortunately, the concept they have about cancer is that it is directly associated with death. I wanted them to see me alive and well with my long hair, nice skin tone and radiant look. I knew that once I started with my first surgery and treatment it was going to be very difficult for me to see them for several months. I knew I wouldn't be able to travel for some time and due to their old age they wouldn't be able to visit me in Miami. That was a hard thing to deal with because throughout the years we've always spent holidays together and I always made it a point to travel to see them with my children at every opportunity. I was able to get a flight for that afternoon. I called my aunt Tere, a very dear person to me, and asked her if she could pick me up at the airport. I didn't give her any details about the reason for my trip and she, being the lady that she is, did not ask any questions.

After making my reservation, I packed my bag and called Tom, who was with the children, to tell him that I needed to talk to him regarding my diagnosis. At that time they were boating on Biscayne Bay, so they came to pick me up at the Marina next to my house. I got on the boat and held my children really tight without saying a word. I was devastated. I was wearing my dark glasses so they wouldn't see my swollen eyes. The mere thought of not being able to see them growing up frightened me. I tried to contain my tears, but I was very sensitive. Even though I was trying to be very strong in front of them, it was very difficult. They both asked me what the doctor had told me about the lump I had on my breast. Tom asked me the same question, but before I started talking to him I decided to talk to my children at their level and in Spanish, which is our language. I explained to them that the tumor was a bad tumor called cancer and that the doctor told me he had to do surgery to remove it. I told them that after the surgery, he was going to give me some very strong medicine that would cure me so I could be like new again. My daughter Izzy started crying a lot. Seeing her like that broke my heart. She was frightened and kept hugging me very tight as if she was afraid we were no longer going to be together. Tommy, on the other hand, was a little more cautious, but asked me straight out if I was going to die. I took a deep breath and tried to remain calm. I told him that the reality was that I didn't know if I was going to die, but I wanted to promise him that I was going to do everything that I could possibly do to avoid dying because I didn't want to leave them alone. He held me in a very gentle manner and kissed me on the cheek. He hugged Izzy and asked her not to cry anymore. He started telling her that everything was going to be all right. The image of Tommy holding his little sister at that moment is something that I am going to treasure forever, because it taught me how a little boy can have so much love to share with his sister.

I can't help to think how difficult the situation must have been for them at that time. The stability that they were accustomed to throughout their lives with me was falling apart. They became very vulnerable and began to face a new reality in which fear, doubt and uncertainty abounded.

After talking to them, I informed Tom of my diagnosis and reminded him that I didn't have medical insurance. I know that he felt bad for me because, even though we have had our huge differences a few months earlier, he could have been able to help me get my medical insurance but opted not to do it. At that time, like so many others, he told me that he was not going to help me get my insurance due to the fact that I had asked for the divorce because I wanted to be on my own. He told me that I would have to figure out how to get my own insurance. Honestly, I don't think that either one of us would have ever imagined that I would be going through this situation.

It is very difficult to live in this country without having medical insurance because the costs are astronomical. Throughout the years I had been covered by the television union insurance, but at that time my company was on a tight budget. When our shows were cancelled without warning, I had to cut expenses and decided to stop paying my medical insurance until my financial situation was better. At the time of canceling my insurance I thought that the worse thing that could happen to me was to be in a car accident, because in Miami people drive very badly. I had contacted my car insurance sales woman, who told me not to worry because I was covered in case of a car accident. I felt relieved and decided that I should not worry about something going wrong with my health. I would have never imagined that this mistake was already growing inside my body. I never imagined I already had cancer.

After a short conversation in which Tom asked me several questions, he agreed to take care of the children while I flew down to Mexico to talk to my grandparents. I knew that I had to take the trip even though it was going to be difficult because they needed to learn about my situation from me and not from somebody else.

I said goodbye to my children and left them on the boat with their dad, telling them repeatedly that I loved them more than anything in the world. I explained to them that I needed to fly to Mexico City to talk to my grandparents because we were not going to be able to see them for several months. I went home to get my luggage, trying to make some sense of this new reality while packing … it was very difficult.

I was closing my suitcase when my friend Rey, who didn't know of the results, stopped by to visit. He brought me a book that he had read, thinking it would be very interesting to me. Since we became friends we have shared several books because we both love to read. As soon as he handed me the book, my eyes felt teary again because it was a story about Lance Armstrong, the American cyclist that had won the Tour de France after conquering testicular cancer. I was totally surprised that this book came into my hands just at the right time. At that moment I told him what was going on with my life. He was totally surprised because he could never have imagined it.

On my way to the airport that afternoon, I was totally exhausted and felt tightness in my chest just thinking about going back to my own city carrying with me this huge sadness.

I spent the almost three hours that it took to fly to Mexico reading the book, which I found very interesting.

It taught me that you must have determination to fight this illness. I was so immersed in reading it, that the flight seemed short. The only problem I had was when I reached the section that talked about chemotherapy. I couldn't read but the first paragraph and had to close it and put it beside me. What I read was scary because I wasn't ready to deal with all of that. I decided to take a break and walk around the plane before I could resume reading the next chapter.

That night in Mexico I talked to my aunt and uncle, who had come to pick me up at the airport. They felt sorry for me. I saw a good side of my uncle that I didn't know before, because right there he offered to take care of my children's school tuition while I was going through the problem, which was a great help for a single mother. They felt the pain that I was facing with this situation, offering me all of their support. My aunt opened up her heart and gave me a lot of love during this whole process.

The next morning I went to my grandparent's house. They were totally surprised to see me in Mexico because they had no idea that I was going to be there. Throughout the years I had surprised them on several occasions, showing up at their house for my grandfather's birthday. Somehow, this time they had a feeling that this was not a regular visit. It can be called intuition, sixth sense or maternal instinct, but upon seeing me my grandmother immediately knew that something was terribly wrong. A week prior to my visit I had told her about the tumor that I had found in my breast. That is why as soon as she saw me in Mexico she knew that I must have been having a problem. At that moment I saw fear in her eyes.

After saying hello and hugging each other, my grandfather stood up from his seat at the table where he was having breakfast and simply said goodbye to us, saying that it was late and he had to go to work. I looked at him with disbelief and asked him to take his seat again, because I needed to tell him of the reason for my trip. At first he didn't want to sit down. He kept looking at his watch. He finally sat down as I explained my problem, all the while trying to be strong and brave and to avoid crying.

As soon as I mentioned the word cancer, my grandmother started crying. She took out some tissue from her dress and kept looking at me, repeating out loud, "It's not possible, not to you." My grandfather, on the other hand, simply told me, "This is a difficult situation, you need to resolve it. I'm going to work, see you this afternoon." He wore his coat, put his hands in his pockets, and started whistling while Jaime, his driver, held on to his briefcase and walked him to the car to take him to his office. My grandfather has always been a great example in my life. He's always offered me support. I know that his reaction that day was simply to block from his mind something painful and difficult. From that day on something very strange happened to him. In a certain way, he decided to deny my illness and to this day hasn't accepted it. It's interesting how the human mind functions when trying to avoid something that causes pain. He and I have always had a great relationship. Even though I am his granddaughter and not his daughter, ever since I can recall, he has called me daughter. He has taken care of me. He has protected me. He has loved me. He has been beside me during my wacky moments. He has always been by my side and by my children's side. It has caused me a great deal of pain to know how much he has suffered due to my illness.

After my grandfather left the house, I didn't know what to do because I had to comfort my grandmother. She was crying non-stop. I kept telling her that everything was going to be all right, but she just kept repeating how worried she was. I hugged her and told her about the great doctors and medicine in the United States. As an example, I used the book that I had been reading on the plane. I, myself, was very afraid, but it was very hard for me to see her, an elderly woman, so worried about her grandchild. We have always had a close relationship. She started to feel that because of being so far apart she was not going to be able to take care of my children or me.

That afternoon I was resting in one of their bedrooms. Suddenly, my grandmother told me that my dad was on the phone wanting to speak to me because he had found out about the diagnosis through one of my brothers. Because our relationship had always been very distant, my initial reaction was one of fear. It had been very difficult for me throughout the years to understand and accept the cold relationship that existed between us. Since I was a little girl I felt rejected by him. I had fought against it during my whole life. Even in my adult life and with my children, I had tried to get close to him, but always found a cold, strict man who had no interest in us. Somehow, the very few times that we saw each other throughout the years, he would make it a point to make me feel that I wasn't good enough to be his daughter. On many occasions he would verbally attack me so that I felt like his enemy more than his daughter did, but the reality is that I have never understood why. When my grandmother told me that my dad was on the phone and wanted to talk to me, I didn't want to it pick up because I was afraid to talk with him. What could he possibly tell me? For a moment I thought about not answering the call because I was sure he was going to attack me emotionally. But being at my grandparent's house and right next to her, I had no choice but to talk to him.

The phone call was not positive at all. It began by him ordering me to give him an explanation and a report about my diagnosis. Then, he went on to tell me that I had brought it upon myself due to the way of life that I was living in Miami. He ended up telling me that I had gotten it through contact with other people. I was listening to him in disbelief and started crying because his words were hurting me in a very profound way, especially because at that time the last thing I needed was more aggression. I continued to listen to him but couldn't even say a word because I was crying out loud. My feelings were an odd mixture of pain, anger and incredulity. I decided not to respond to him. I simply let him finish everything he had to say, told him that I understood, and said goodbye. Previous to that conversation, we hadn't spoken to each other in more than a year. I thought to myself that I would be better off without any further communication between us. I went back to my room where my grandparents were waiting for me. They both realized that the phone call had hurt me deeply. I sat down at the edge of the bed. They were both hugging me, telling me to try to understand him and that his reaction was his own way of showing that he cared about me.

The following morning my father phoned my grandparents' home again. He spoke only with my grandmother, telling her that he would have me flown over to Texas to get a second opinion. He had decided he wanted to take me to the hospital that he and my grandparents had attended frequently throughout the years because the doctors there had his absolute trust. He wanted to make sure that I would get the best diagnosis possible. When my grandmother told me this, I looked at her with disbelief. At first I thought that my dad simply wanted to become the hero saving the fallen daughter. I was under the impression that he had never cared about my health. He practically didn't know my children. From the time I first left home, he never helped me financially, not even in my most difficult situations. It was hard for me to understand that after so many years, he was going to use his money and time to help me out. The truth is that it was very difficult for me to believe it, so I talked about it with my grandmother. She insisted that after all, he was my father and I needed to let him help me and guide me. I was totally confused.

After having breakfast, my father called again to talk to me. His tone of voice was less aggressive than before, sounding more at ease. He asked me to go with him to Texas to seek a second opinion, offering to cover all of my expenses because he knew of my financial situation. I thought to myself that, since he was taking care of the bill, I had nothing to lose and yet a lot to win if I took advantage of the trip to get some of the exams that Doctor D. had required. I was grateful for his offer. I was honest with him from that moment on by telling him that, even though I would go with him to Texas for a second opinion, I had made the decision to receive treatment in Miami because I wanted to be with my children throughout this whole process. I wanted to be very direct to avoid misunderstandings as far as what I was going to do with my life. I told him and everybody that I wasn't pretending to be a martyr, but that I was a very determined woman ready to fight with everything I had to try to overcome this illness for my own good and for the good of my children. Finally, we agreed to see each other in Texas the following week.

That morning, while I was reading at my grandparent's house, my Aunt Tere called to say that her mother wanted to talk to me. Her mother is a woman whom I have seen throughout the years at weddings, parties and family reunions, but with whom I really never had a close relationship. To a certain extent, I was surprised that she had wanted to talk to me. Tere told me that her mother wanted to share with me something that she had lived through that was similar to what I was facing. She picked me up and took me to her mother's house.

Doña Enriqueta is a beautiful, very distinguished and elegant woman, whom I have always admired because of the way she always takes care of herself. I was under the impression that she had always lived an easy life, full of parties and social engagements, without any major worries. I knew very little about her private life. When she told me that she previously had cancer of the lymph nodes, I was totally surprised. During a couple of hours she talked to me about her experience and how difficult it had been for her. She was married and her three children were teenagers at the time. In those days, medical problems were treated with a lot of discretion and people didn't really have the support group of family and friends that we can count on today. Her story inspired me tremendously—even though our family and financial situations, diagnoses and treatments were different—because for the first time I realized that I wasn't alone with this problem and that cancer can attack anybody. I felt privileged that she had shared her experience with me. Because of her words I knew that I needed to be strong and face the situation with dignity, just like she had done in her time. Her story seemed very touching to me since I knew her for years and never even suspected that she could have faced something like this before. Thanks to that conversation, I understood the value of communication and the value of information. When somebody that has lived with this problem can share it with somebody that is beginning to confront it, it can have a strong influence in the way that person starts facing the situation. Seeing that she was so sure of herself, so strong and so dignified, while reliving something as difficult, personal and fragile, gave me the strength to start facing my situation. At that moment I realized that something as difficult as cancer can create a chain of love and support between two women of different generations. Her melancholy while telling me of her situation, life, fears, fights, suffering and sheer will to forge ahead for her own children's sake were to me like an injection of enthusiasm, faith, determination and strength. Thanks to that conversation, I was able to erect the pillars upon which I would build my fight throughout this Difficult Journey.

That same afternoon, after being really touched by the conversation, I knew saying goodbye to my grandparents would be very difficult. My grandmother, who by nature is a very cold woman, started crying, breaking my heart. My grandfather seemed really worried. I wish I could have avoided causing them so much pain, but it was due to a situation totally out of my hands. The emotions that we felt at that moment are difficult to explain because, to a certain extent, the word cancer is a death sentence and the thought of perhaps never seeing each other again crossed our minds more than once. Even though I wanted to keep a positive attitude, the fear that cancer instills is huge. It is a very difficult feeling to express.

That evening I flew back to Miami. I was happy to be home with my children. I hugged them and kissed them. I explained to them that during my trip to Mexico I had come to realize that a lot of people truly loved us and were very supportive of us. After finishing our prayers, Izzy looked at me. With some fear and in her tender voice, she asked me if I knew then that I was going to die. One more time I didn't have the right answer for her. I didn't want to lie to her, but once again promised her that I was going to try to fight to stay alive, telling her that only God knows when it's our time to leave. That was a very emotional evening and, as a special concession, I let them sleep in the bed with me.

When I went back to my house, city and familiar surroundings, I felt new sensations. Even though I was tired from the trip and the strong emotions I had experienced, I started to realize that in the most difficult time new doors always open and good souls appear along the way to guide and bring some light to us.

From those early days with the disease, life began to teach me great lessons about compassion, kindness, generosity, love and tenderness. And from the very beginning I knew that I had to appreciate, understand, accept and learn from it.

SECOND OPINION

Before going to Texas for a second opinion, my life became filled with chaos during the few days that I was in Miami. The phone rang constantly with calls from people who were just finding out about my illness. Everybody kept asking me the same questions. I talked to the director of my children's school to ask him to pay special attention to their behavior and moods. I needed to know if either he or any of the teachers noticed changes in their grades so that we could deal with it in the best possible way. I am aware that when the fundamental structure of a child's life is altered, it can affect their state of mind and behavior. What my children were facing at that time wasn't easy.

The news of my diagnosis was surprising to him. Right away, teachers and parents started talking to us, offering their support and prayers. Every time that I took my children to school, someone stopped me to cheer me up. I received offers to help take my children from and to school. Parents whom I never socialized with before would stop me to talk, either to relate a story about someone that was going through something similar or just to say we were on their minds. I wasn't looking for extra attention for my children simply because I had cancer. I wanted to make sure that they had somebody they could count on, especially on days that they were particularly sad, confused or afraid. I believe that when your fundamental life changes at home during childhood, school becomes your refuge.

When the time came for me to go to Texas, I didn't like the idea of going alone with my father, just the two of us. Due to our lack of contact previously, I didn't know what we could possibly talk about, what his mood with me would be, if he was really going to help and support me, or if he simply wanted to feel less guilty about the lack of a relationship between us. It is very strange to write this, but I believe that he was one of the people who knew me the least. The thought of spending three days together with so much tension between us was a little uncomfortable for me.

Anyway, once I decided to take the trip I tried to look at it in a positive way despite the difficulty of the situation. It made me feel good to think that at least this time my father was concerned about me because it was a feeling that I hadn't felt before.

The day of my trip arrived. During the flight I was constantly worrying about those three days. I was not only worried about cancer, but also about spending time with him, although I was very grateful that he was taking some of his time to take me to the hospital. They diverted my flight to New Orleans and after a couple of hours we flew into San Antonio. My father was right outside the gate waiting for me. I saw him, smiled at him and kissed him. He looked at me and the first thing he told me was that the eyeglasses I was wearing were pretty awful. He asked me if I really needed them to see or if I just liked wearing them. I felt a little uncomfortable with his comment, not only since I really need them to see but also because I thought they were nice! But at that time I knew that the fact that he was trying to make an effort to help me didn't change the fact that my dad was my dad and wasn't going to change his behavior towards me. I decided not to let his comments hurt me but simply to ignore them.

We picked up my luggage and started driving to the hospital that was about an hour and a half away by car. During the whole ride there, we only spoke about trivial issues such as the weather, the landscape and the traffic. We stopped to have dinner at a restaurant across the street from the medical center just across from our hotel. After eating we walked into the hotel and registered. It was late at night and we were both tired from the trip. My father had reserved two rooms, one for each one of us. I felt relieved when I found out about our sleeping arrangements because I thought that way I would have some privacy to cry alone.

The next morning we got up before dawn and registered at the hospital to start with the tests. Assuming that I was going to be receiving the same diagnosis as in Miami, I brought with me the X-rays, the ultrasound and the biopsy results so we wouldn't have to repeat those. Along with those, I also brought the prescriptions for the new tests that Doctor D., my oncologist in Miami, had ordered. I had asked my father if it was OK to have them done there since he was going to take care of the expenses. Without those exams they couldn't operate on me in Miami.

When you are living under those circumstances, days pass by very slowly, with the fear and the anguish that the cancer continues to grow in your body. That is why I wanted to get the most done during this trip since I would not be leaving the hospital for three days.

I noticed that my dad was worried about my situation and the feeling I had about this was a little strange. On one hand I felt sorry to see him that concerned and anguished. On the other, it felt good to know that he was worried about me and I was happy to have him next to me.

Between tests and analyses, we had some long periods of silence while sitting in the respective waiting rooms. That's where I started reading all the information I could find about cancer. I tried to spend my free time busy so the wait wouldn't be as tenuous. Every time I read something new, I'd share it with my father. Even though I was feeling that he was trying to support me emotionally, all those years of lack of communication and absence of a relationship cannot be erased overnight. Although we were both trying to make an effort to ease the situation, you could still feel a lot of tension between us.

During the first few hours of exams, he would insist that cancer was contagious and that I had gotten it because of the way he thought I was living. I know that he didn't really mean it because he is a very well educated man. That is why I want to believe that it was his way of showing his anger and frustration, trying to blame someone or something for the situation. Mentally, I was very well prepared not to let his comments hurt me or affect me. I decided to view his words as merely the reflection of a fearful and anguished father.

As soon as we had our first meeting with the doctor, I asked him for an explanation of the factors that can cause this kind of cancer. Although I was a little bit apprehensive, I asked him directly if there was a remote possibility that someone had given it to me. After this question, the doctor looked at us with disbelief because our appearance would lead one to believe that we were well-educated people who should know that cancer is not contagious. Even so, he reiterated it several times.

The doctor needed to examine me and asked my father to leave the room for a moment. That's when I talked to the doctor, explaining that my father was very worried about my condition and had never approved of me living in

Miami away from my family. That's why he was using this excuse to try to make me believe that I was somehow being punished for not continuing the family tradition of living at home. The doctor understood that it was simply a family situation. When my father came back into his office, he told us repeatedly that there is absolutely no way that a person can get cancer from another person. I felt relieved.

That same day, my youngest brother Migue met with us at the hospital to spend the day with us. I was very happy to see him because during the previous year we had grown apart. The fact that he was there made the situation with my dad a little less tense.

After three days of tests, X-rays and a wide variety of analyses, we were finally ready to go see the last oncologist to get the final diagnosis. All of the doctors' conclusions, from the internist to the radiologist to the pathologist, were the same as those that I received in Miami. My father and I assumed that the visit with the last oncologist was going to be no different. Early that morning before leaving the hotel, we packed our bags assuming that we were leaving as soon as we received the last diagnosis. We walked into the oncologist's office. After the usual wait, the oncologist met with the two of us. His assistant was with him at all times. He started pulling out papers and X-rays, confirming the breast cancer diagnosis. He explained to us the possibility that there was already metastasis. He told us that the only way to know the full extent of the damage was to have my lymph nodes removed and analyzed. I was a little bit relieved to find out that the diagnosis in Texas was exactly the same as the one I got from Doctor D. in Miami. At least I knew that the opinions were the same in both places and the procedure to follow was practically the same. I was pleased to hear that all the doctors emphasized that the treatment should take place close to home because it was going to be long and difficult and I needed to try to keep stability in my surroundings and life. All of sudden, the doctor stood up, turned on the X-ray light and, looking directly at me, told me with a very serious voice, "Everything is the same. However, I am very sorry to tell you that we have found a tumor in the left kidney and it seems to us that it is cancerous. The complication here is that the metastasis from breast cancer does not go to the kidneys, but to the lungs, the bones and the brain, so we firmly believe that we have to deal with another different kind of cancer. It is our opinion that the first thing that should be done is an operation to remove the tumor and have it analyzed. The reason is that kidney biopsies can generate incorrect readings since large masses or tumors such as this can be invaded with cancerous cells only in certain places. This can make it possible during the biopsy for the needle to enter where there are no cancerous cells, leading us to believe that the tumor is benign when in reality it is not."

While I was listening to the doctor my world started to collapse again, only this time my father was with me and I could see fear in his eyes. I knew that I needed to be strong, but it was very difficult. This diagnosis caught me completely off guard. Pretending to be very interested in the appearance of my tumor, I stood up from my chair and proceeded to observe the X-ray to have the doctor show me exactly what he was talking about. I have no idea how to read X-rays, but I guess I was trying to look for a way to avoid the problem or at least gain some time to let the news sink in. Looking at the X-ray, all I saw was a big ball covering the left side of my left kidney. I didn't need to be a doctor to be able to see the difference between the two kidneys.

Once again I didn't know what to do. I was totally confused and worried. I wanted to cry but I knew I needed to control myself in front of my father. Right there, the oncologist ordered some new tests because they had also found some suspicious spots on my lungs and certain parts of my spinal chord. He told us again that he was sorry about the results, indicating we should go back with the head doctor that had new information about my case.

Every time I looked at my dad, I couldn't help but feel bad. He was so worried. To a certain extent, the same thing extent that happened to my grandmother and me in Mexico was happening between my father and me. I needed to be the strong one. I needed to console him because I could see that this was too much for him to handle.

There was nothing we could do except follow the doctor's instructions. Our plans to go home that day had to be cancelled and we simply started with another day of tests, X-rays and analyses.

That night was very difficult for both of us. We went out to have a nice dinner and tried to make small talk about the food, the wine and the restaurant. Somehow we avoided both talking about the illness. My father kept repeating constantly that those were very good doctors, that they were the very best in the world, and that I should consider the possibility of having them operate and treat me instead of doing it in Miami.

The following morning we made our last round at the hospital. We met with the specialists, who gave us their final diagnosis. Luckily, they had found nothing more and the other spots in my lung and bones did not seem to be cancerous, so we could return home. We both tried to pretend that we were totally calm, but we knew that inside our minds there was turmoil. We said goodbye to the doctors and their support staff. We were going back to our homes with this bad news, but at least we had a second opinion and the difficulty of my situation was clear.

We drove from the hospital to the airport. The ride was long and silent. Every now and then we would talk, but I kept staring through the window. Tears were rolling constantly from my eyes. I tried very hard to not let my father see me crying. I was feeling so much pain I wanted to scream. I wanted to run away from it all. I wanted to get on my flight, go back home, spend time with my kids, and make decisions. I needed my own time and space to try to make sense of the situation. I needed to be alone to think, meditate and create a connection with my inner self. I thought I was facing a difficult situation when I was diagnosed with breast cancer, but now I felt devastated. I needed to think.

Almost at the end of the trip my father asked me to go back home and think very hard about what I was going to do. He offered his emotional support and some financial support, but with some strings attached. To tell the truth, at that point I was starting to get tired of relatives offering me some kind of conditional help. I told him that I was very grateful to him, but that I needed to think of my children and not just myself and didn't want to create anymore confusion in their lives, so I was going to be treated near my home. I asked him to please respect my decision because he needed to understand that nobody was more interested in my own health than me.

After a long silence, he offered once again his emotional support during that Difficult Journey. At that moment, I found a new meaning to my illness. By divine intervention, closeness between my father and me was beginning to emerge. That was something that I had envisioned during many years. It was happening at last.

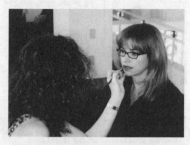
Getting ready to shoot my new pilot the day I found the lump.

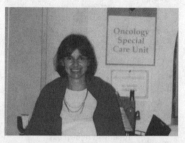
I never thought I would be a patient at the oncology unit at that age.

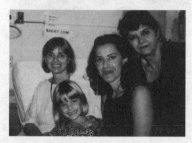
After my first set of three surgeries with my mom, my sister and my daughter.

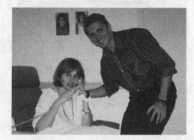
Antonio visiting me at the hospital.

I started loosing my hair so I had to go bold.

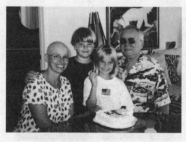
With my father and my children.

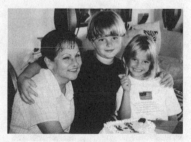
Tommy and Izzi with Adela.

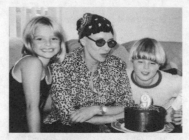

Tommy's 9th birthday.

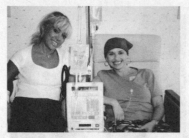

Getting my chemo with my friend Lilia.

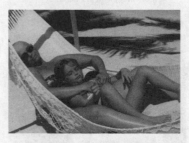

Enjoying some quiet time with Izzy.

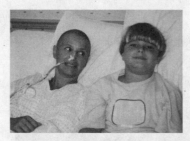

Even though I looked pretty bad kept fighting.

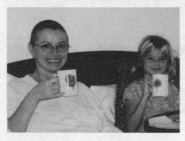

Enjoying a cup of tea with Izzy.

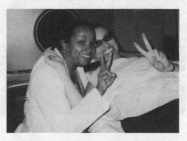

Getting ready to receive my radiation treatment.

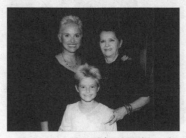

Three generations: with my mother and my daughter.

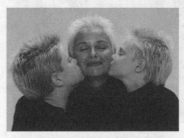

Love is what moves the world. Here I am with my children.

SURGERIES

"My mommy had to go to the hospital to have surgeries. I was very, very worried. My little sister Izzy was crying a lot because my mommy had to be in the hospital for many days. I was very worried and couldn't sleep at night, but during the day my friends at school made me feel real good because they would ask about my mom everyday. While she was in the hospital, Izzy and I went to visit her almost everyday and brought her flowers, letters that we wrote to her, and some necklaces that we made at home."

— Tommy

Upon returning to Miami from Texas, my main concern was to make an appointment to see Doctor D., my oncologist, again. I needed to give him the results of all the tests. I got an appointment to see him. On the way to his office, something really strange happened to me. I lost my voice. That's right! Completely lost my voice. I was mute. I couldn't say even one word. It was a horrible feeling. While I was at his office, I had this terrible sensation of helplessness because, besides trying desperately to communicate with him everything I was feeling, I had returned home full of questions and doubts after my diagnosis in Texas. I didn't have any voice, which did not allow me to ask or tell him anything. The harder I tried to speak, the more frustrating it became and the more anguish it created.

Doctor D., with his patience and experience, kept telling me not to worry because he saw it as a result of the stress that I was going through. So he prescribed some drops and a lot of rest, assuring me that my voice would come back within a couple of days.

I needed to talk to him about the tumor on my kidney. I wanted to know his opinion about it and have him refer me to a renal oncologist. With a little bit of sign language and by writing on a piece of paper, he understood what I was saying. We got a hold of our friend Tito, the pathologist. After a short conversation between them, they decided who would be the best doctor to treat this problem. Taking into consideration my financial situation, Doctor D. suggested that the kidney surgery should be done at the same time as the breast and lymph node surgeries. He told me that, even though recuperating from three surgeries was going to be more painful and difficult, financially I was going to be better off having to pay only once for the operating room, anesthesiologist, nurses, recovery room, intensive care unit, etc. To tell the truth, this doctor has been a real angel along the way because, for the first time in my life, I found a doctor that truly loves his career and is conscientious about the financial situation of his patients. Besides helping me by suggesting doing the surgeries at the same time, one day he walked into my hospital room and gave me the business card of the person in charge of financial aid through a charity service from the hospital. He urged me to contact her to explain my situation and try to get some help. If it weren't because of him, I would have never known that the possibility of help was available. With all his caring and interest, he showed that he looked at me as a real person and not just a number. Even though I have written him thank you notes and my children have made him some drawings to display in his office, I can never get tired of being grateful to him for everything he did for me. He showed me the dedication, compassion and respect that he has for his career by letting me know that there are still some doctors that truly practice medicine out of love and not just for the sake of making money.

That day I left the doctor's office with tears in my eyes again. By then I think I had the cleanest liver in the whole city—there is a tale that says that the liver is cleansed through the release of tears. Even though I have cried my whole life, during this time I was extremely sensitive and tears would just roll down my face at the slightest thing.

It was rather unusual that I went to his office all by myself. But deep down inside of me, I was feeling that my days of independence were coming to an end, at least temporarily, and I was feeling a great need to take care of myself on my own.

One of the most tiring issues during the whole process of the illness was the constant phone calls. Although I knew that they were from those who loved me and worried about me, it got to a point that so many calls were making me feel uneasy or tired because everybody wanted the same answers and I was forced to repeat the same story over and over again. I am very grateful to everybody that was concerned, but as soon as I started feeling weak I decided to limit the amount calls I could take each day. At that time, my mother and brother's constant calls to me, asking about the date for my surgeries, became very difficult. I didn't have much to tell them because the dates did not depend on me but on the doctors, even though I understood that they needed to find reasonable airfares in order to come and be with me. It got to a point that they unknowingly made me feel bad because I didn't have an answer, so I decided to not take any more calls from them until I had a set date.

One afternoon I was at home when I got a call about an appointment to see a renal oncologist. They gave it to me with eight days' notice. So I called my mother to tell her about it and asked her if she could come and spend some time with us since, after her initial reaction, she had offered to do so. She proposed to stay with me while I had the surgeries in order to help me a little bit at home. Although I didn't yet know a date for the surgeries, I assumed it was going to be a few days after my visit to the renal oncologist.

My mother arrived at Miami the day before my doctor's appointment. She went with me to that initial visit. Upon meeting the doctor, I thought he looked extremely young to have as much experience as his colleagues had told me. Truthfully, his short height and baby face made me question if he was as professional and expert as they had told me. I think he read my mind when I was thinking about it because all of a sudden he started telling me that he wasn't as young as he seemed, assuring me that these types of surgeries were common to him. I felt relieved once he told me that. He took a look at my X-rays and did a physical exam. His diagnosis was just as the doctor's in Texas. The tumor was cancerous, encapsulated, and had the typical characteristics of cancer. He then explained to me that he was going to try to do a partial kidney surgery, removing the tumor and half of the kidney instead of the entire kidney. It's called a partial nephrectomy. He wasn't sure that he was going to be able to do it because he needed to open me up to see the exact size of the tumor and determine where it had expanded. Only then could he make the determination. I felt relieved when he told me that he agreed with Doctor D. in coordinating the surgeries, making it entirely up to them to find a day in which they could both operate on me.

The waiting time between the diagnosis and the coordination of both doctors to determine the dates was agonizing. On the one hand, I couldn't stop thinking that the cancer was spreading inside my body without being able to do anything to stop it. But on the other, I knew that everything was outside my control and there was nothing I could do to accelerate the process. I had called the secretaries of both doctors several times to ask about the date of the surgery. I kept feeling that they were in no hurry to find a date. Days went by and I grew more impatient. I called the doctors' offices again on a Thursday afternoon. After asking the same question about the date, I was told that the operation would have to wait for at least two months because the doctors' schedules were conflicting. When I heard that I felt terrible. I couldn't believe it and got really angry with the woman who had told me. I was so upset that I raised my voice to her. My frustration was huge. I asked her for at least a moment to put herself in my shoes so that she could understand how difficult it was for me to live each day knowing that I had cancer and that there was nothing I could do to try to save myself. I told her that I was very frustrated because it seemed that this huge problem that I was facing seemed like something trivial to all of them. I broke down over the phone with her. I guess she felt sorry for me because she told me that she understood my pain and she was going to try to do something to help me. We hung up the phone. About half an hour later she called me back to tell me that she herself had spoken to both doctors and that they were willing to do the surgeries that same Saturday, two days later. I thought that it was rather soon, but I was very excited because I didn't want to live anymore with the agony of waiting.

My youngest brother Migue and my sister Veronica flew out the next day to be with me. It was interesting because, of all of my siblings, they were the ones that I didn't expect to see next to me, since I didn't have a close relationship with either of them. I was happy to see them, knowing at the same time that they had come to be me because they were afraid that I wasn't going to make it. Although I had called my dad to ask him to be with me, he told me that he wasn't going to come because my mother was with me and their relationship is not cordial. I was hurt by his attitude. In a situation like the one I was living, I needed the support and care of both my parents and didn't like the fact that they had to make me choose which one of the two was going to be with me. Since their divorce, there had been a lot of tension between them, but at that particular time I needed their moral support, not their personal issues.

I spent the whole day Friday at the hospital doing some analyses and last minute tests, along with pre-registering. By nighttime I wasn't able to sleep. I was nervous, worried and afraid. I kept wondering what the doctors were going to find. I was worried about my children. The next morning Tom came to pick them up and take them to his house for the weekend. I had asked him to do so, thinking that it was the best for them because by being removed from the problem they would at least forget about it a little bit. Saying goodbye to them that morning before going to the hospital was very difficult because the three of us were worried. After hugging and kissing them, and praying together, they took off. I got ready to go to the hospital. I really didn't have anything with me except for X-rays and test results. Before leaving my house, I went back to my room one last time, meditated, and prayed on my own in silence. I prayed from the bottom of my heart, asking God and my guardian angels to do with my life what was best. I had mixed feelings. On the one hand, I had the feeling that somehow things were going to work out OK. On the other, in looking at my prognosis, I knew great risks existed. It was a difficult situation because even up to the time that I arrived at the operating room I didn't know if I was going to come out of the surgery with or without my breast or with or without my kidney.

In addition to my brother, sister and mother, Antonio came to the house that morning to go with us to the hospital. It amazes me the strong spiritual bond that ties us together. His company and unconditional support made me feel safe, as if nothing bad could happen to me. From the moment I met him, I felt a strong connection. Even though we are not a couple, we complement each other in a very special way. His presence by my side has reinforced my belief in the reincarnation of the souls, because I have always felt that we have shared previous lives and experiences. He complains a lot about me, telling me constantly that I am "that cross" that life has put in front of him, but I know that he loves me just as much as I love him.

At the hospital, the time had come to walk into the pre-operating room where I was only allowed to have two visitors with me. I said goodbye to Antonio. My mother decided to wait outside so that my brother and sister could be with me. I walked to the nurse's station to confirm my identity. The nurses couldn't believe that my bracelet indicated it was the day of my birthday. They all started making comments such as, "Good way to celebrate your birthday." In reality, my birthday wasn't that day but four days later; they had made a typo.

I lay flat on the stretcher wearing my hospital robe as they hooked me up to the IV. Shortly after my two doctors came to say hello to me, they explained exactly what they were going to do. To my surprise, the kidney surgery was going to be the first one because the tumor was on my left kidney and they needed to position me on my right side for the surgery. This made matters a little complicated since the breast tumor and the lymph nodes were on my right side. They had to tilt the operating table in a manner so that Doctor D. could operate on those areas without putting my weight on the left side. I was definitely afraid, scared and nervous when the anesthesiologist came to talk to me. I asked him repeatedly if he was absolutely sure that he was going to be able to keep me unconscious during the whole time. I explained to him that I was going to have three surgeries, and the idea of waking up between them frightened me. I think that the fear of feeling pain while I was having the surgery was more than if I was just to wake up during the surgery, but he asked me to relax and trust him because, "He had a lot of experience putting women to sleep." His comment made me laugh. It was during that conversation that I thought I heard a familiar voice talking to the nurses. I raised my head a little bit and was able to see Juan talking to them. He had come to say goodbye to me. With his good looks, he had managed to get all the way to the pre-operating room. I was glad to see him. After his usual scolding—according to him I gave him the wrong directions to get to the hospital—he held my hand, kissed my lips, and told me that he wouldn't let me go to surgery without first seeing and talking to me. I was very excited to see him by my side. He kept holding my hand and caressing my hair until the nurse came to take me to the operating room. He then grasped my hand tightly and softly whispered into my ear, "I love you." I looked into his eyes, gave him a smile, and said to him, "I know."

I don't remember anything about the surgeries because the anesthesia had worked just as the anesthesiologist told me it would. The only thing I remember is waking up angry and afraid because in my mind I thought they had only performed the first surgery and I needed to go back to have the other two. I remember that I kept asking the anesthesiologist to explain to me why the anesthesia was wearing off if they still had work to do. I think the nurses and doctors are used to these types of reactions from patients because they wouldn't pay much attention to me. They simply went about doing their work. I kept raising my voice, asking the same thing over and over again until the anesthesiologist finally came to my side, asking me to relax and explaining that all of the surgeries had been done and that I was already in the recovery room. Although I had no notion of the time that had passed, I had been in the operating room for almost nine hours. During the first few hours of my recovery, I woke up several times with the same anguish but, as soon as the nurse would ask me to relax because the surgeries were over, I would just go back to sleep.

Several hours later I woke up while they were wheeling my bed down the hall to my room. The hallways were very bright and bothered my eyes. All of a sudden, I heard a lot of people talking all around me. I was still sedated and couldn't even open my eyes. I felt very confused and didn't really know what was going on. Suddenly, I heard Antonio's voice whispering in my ear. He was saying everything was all right and that it seemed like the kidney tumor had no cancer. I remember opening my eyes right at that moment, seeing his huge smile full of happiness. In a strange way and at the same time, I felt the presence of a white angel wrapping his wings around me and giving me the good news. Then, I found myself like in a cloud of white light where the huge white wings were covering my whole body and protecting me. I don't know if that was a dream, a vision, or a hallucination due to the anesthesia, but that's exactly what I felt. The feeling was very real. At that moment I didn't even have the strength to talk. I simply let him hold my hand and smiled at him. I was very happy with the news and very grateful to the universe.

Looking at it from a spiritual point of view, I honestly believe that during the surgeries my protective angels were present. From the scientific point of view, it is difficult to believe that two oncologists who were specialists in kidney tumors could have diagnosed my tumor as cancerous when it was not. I wasn't the only one shocked by the news. Even the doctors were surprised. I choose to believe that from heaven they helped to make my problem smaller, because if this tumor had indeed been cancerous a totally different course of action would have been required to fight two very different kinds of cancer. I am convinced that the many people who prayed for me in their own way and the positive energy of all those people made it possible that my angels transformed the bad into good so that I could recover my health easier. I have no way to prove this, but I choose to believe that this happened because I like feeling protected by the universe.

After leaving the recovery room, they took me to a private room inside the oncology department's intensive care unit (ICU). I hardly remember the first couple of days in ICU because I was too sedated to be able to tolerate the pain. What I do remember with a lot of fondness is that every time I opened my eyes I saw flowers and more flowers in my room, which made me feel happy. I felt the constant presence of my friends around me, surrounding me with love. Marco, one of my twin brothers, arrived on the second day. I remember feeling very happy that he had made the trip because it had been at least three years since I last saw him. During those first days, I missed my children and wanted to have them close to me. I knew that for them it would be very difficult to see me hooked up to so many IVs, so I decided to wait until the third day after surgery to see them in my room.

During my stay at the hospital, my brothers took turns keeping me company at night and helped caring for my children during the day. Tommy and Izzy came to see me on the third day, bringing along a beautiful flower arrangement and some necklaces that they had made at home. Izzy also brought me several love letters that she had written to me. I had asked my sister to stick my children's pictures on the wall right in front of my bed because I somehow wanted to feel their presence in the room with me at all times. After reading Izzy's letters, we also placed them on the wall so that everybody could read them. Doctors and nurses would come into my room just to read the beautiful phrases she had written: "Mommy, I hope you recover soon so that we can go shopping forever," "Mommy, I love you very much and hope you never have cancer again," "Mommy, I hope you recover so we can be together always and go to Spain together."

Hospital rooms tend to be very cold but, somehow, you could feel love, positive energy and good feelings in my room. The flower arrangements that kept coming constantly were a reminder that there was a world of friends outside of that room who were thinking of me and wishing me well. The love that I began to feel during those days is still with me and will be forever. I have learned that one reaps what one has sown. When someone lives at peace and is happy, it projects outwardly to the rest of the people and comes back to you. In this sense, I can say that I am a very fortunate person because life has taught me what sincere love is all about.

I've said repeatedly that my biggest concern at that time was how cancer was going to affect my children. At that age they are so innocent that the simple thought of trying to imagine what a child is feeling when he's worried about losing a parent makes a mother very sad. From the very beginning I decided that I wanted them to be a vital force in my recovery, which is why I waited eagerly for their daily visits to the hospital so that I could go walking with them down the hallways. Like normal kids, they would fight to be the one pushing the mobile IV apparatus. They kept telling me that it was funny how our roles seemed to be reversed because it was them that seemed like the mommy and daddy taking care of their child.

During one of those walks, reality struck when I passed by the sign hanging at the entrance of the unit where I was staying: "Oncology Intensive Care Unit." Even though I had walked by that sign several times during those days, at that particular moment it hit me very hard. It was as if at last I was starting to realize what was happening to me. During several days, that sign kept coming into my mind. It was very difficult for me to comprehend what I was going through. I kept remembering how a month and a half before I was enjoying life to the fullest. Surrounded by my best friends, I was planning a year of exciting triumphs, both personal and professional. Just a month earlier we had taped the pilots of our new TV series and we had assumed that by now we were going to be signing contracts and negotiating productions. Now I felt protected by the hospital walls that, although very green and empty, were welcoming to me. Life can teach a hard lesson and take a sudden change in direction.

During the afternoon of the third day in the hospital I was laying down in my bed, in the company of my mother and sister, when a very elegant lady wearing a blue suit came to see me. She said hello to me very cordially and told me that she was the representative of the billing department from the hospital. She needed to talk to me to arrange how they were going to get paid. She apologized for having to visit me in my room and ask me for money when I had been recently operated on, but she told me that it was her job. I felt very bad because I knew that I didn't have medical insurance and didn't have the money that I owed them. I talked to her honestly telling her that I didn't have the $80,000 that she was asking for at that time, but I gave her my word that I would start making payments as soon as I was able to go back to work. Trying to minimize the importance of the situation, I told her that she didn't need to worry about me because after just having had three surgeries I wasn't going to be able to run away from the hospital on my own. I asked her for the name of the person in charge of her department so that I could go and talk to him or her directly to arrange a method of payment. I promised to stop by her office before leaving the hospital.

Once she left the room, I realized that my mother was very worried because the amount I owed the hospital alone within such a short period of time was extremely high and she wasn't in position to help me financially even if she had wanted to. I, as usual, tried to make the problem seem smaller than it really was so that she wouldn't worry so much. But the reality was that I couldn't even go to sleep, worrying about the fact that I had two young children to support, was very ill, and owed large amounts of money. I was really facing a very difficult situation. The fourth day at the hospital was my real birthday. Although I spent it in a rather unusual way, I had a lot to celebrate because I was alive. That day the telephone did not stop ringing with friends and family calling me to wish me the best. Those calls, as well as the visits, helped make my day go faster and didn't leave a lot of time to dwell on my problems.

In one of the few moments that I had by myself in my room, my friend Tito, the pathologist, walked in with a box of chocolates to wish me a happy birthday. He sat down to talk with me. I told him how worried I was after the visit by the lady from the billing department the day before. He looked at me and with a very peaceful voice told me, "Relax, lady. Problems that can be solved with money are not real problems. Problems are the ones that can't be resolved even if you have all the money in the world; those are the real problems." I have thought a lot about this phrase and finally understand how right he was.

That night I was able to sleep a little bit better because, thanks to Tito's words, I had found new meaning to the value of life and questioned the importance that we sometimes place in irrelevant things throughout our lives. I started to realize that so many times I've been so worried about unnecessary things when the only thing they do is make me waste my energy and strength and that ultimately those problems have never been as bad as I thought they seemed. Eventually, they all had a solution. His comment helped me to understand how money is something created by us humans to which we assign a greater value than it really has, yet health, feelings and love really exist and are capable of breaking barriers, opening doors, and finding more solutions than money can. These feelings have helped me find answers at times when I have been full of uncertainty and doubt because, at the end of the day, these feelings are much stronger than any of the material things you can acquire with money. Thanks to Tito, I was able to look at my financial problem from another perspective because I understood that, as long as I was alive and healthy, I could somehow find the tools that I needed to fight, continue living, supporting my children, and paying my bills.

As of that moment, my healing process had a new perspective. That was when I decided that my priority should be to fight the error that was inside of my cells, repeating constantly to myself that a positive and triumphant attitude was vital to my cure.

TO LIVE AGAIN

"The only good thing about cancer was that it helped us to see how many good friends we have. From the time my mom went into surgery, we always had flowers in the house and our friends always come to visit her and then take us to dinner or swimming in the pool. Sometimes they also bring us gifts."

—*Izzy*

"... our house always smells very nice with so many flowers. Poor mommy, she feels really sick lately, but the phone is always ringing and she always has friends coming by. I liked the fact that now she lets us play to guess words."

—*Tommy*

Six weeks had passed since I left the hospital. Six difficult weeks of recovering at home. Six weeks, during which I had plenty of time to think, sleep, rest, read, enjoy the views from my balcony, and continue with a spiritual quest that began when I started this process. They were six weeks in which my appreciation for life was being modified. Six weeks of changes, internally and externally. Six weeks full of physical pain, especially where I had the incisions from the surgeries. Six weeks of learning to live with my mother again. Six weeks during which my communication with the external world was only by telephone, because I only left the house to go straight to the doctor and back. I was very weak physically and mentally exhausted. I was still trying to comprehend that what was happening to me was real because a lot of times I felt that everything was just a nightmare from which I would eventually wake up.

During several weeks I would spend my days just sitting in a comfortable chair on my balcony contemplating the ocean and looking at the city, asking myself time and time again how much more I had left to discover before I was able to move forward with my life. Those were weeks full of fear and of great emotional and physical vulnerability. During those difficult weeks, I constantly had company. The visits from Juan every single day were very good for me. Almost everyday he would arrive at my house at 10 in the morning to see how I was feeling. He would stay with me, keeping me company and talking with me for several hours. During that time I learned to understand him and to see how all of us are in a constant search to find our own true identity—a search that is different to each one of us and never ends. We would spend hours talking about different topics, not necessarily about work. The love and respect that I always felt towards him was growing every day. He was involved in a very erratic personal relationship, so our morning conversations usually started with his complaints from his life at home. After he let it out, our conversations always turned more philosophical and profound. Thanks to the fact that he was involved in that relationship, I learned another great lesson because I realized that what he felt for me was sincere and without any expectations since he didn't have to spend so much time with me every single day. He did it gladly and with love. I will always remember him fondly for that reason.

One of those days during this time, Sandra came to visit me. She seemed really sad. Although we had known each other for a couple of years, we had never been true friends. That morning she came to talk to me because she needed to get things off her chest and confide in someone about her situation. Perhaps seeing me so weak and in bed I was the appropriate person. Without getting into too many details about her personal life, she confided in me that she was pregnant and, because of the fact that she wasn't married and she already had children, she was not going to be looked on favorably by society. We explored different alternatives. I helped her to realize that, even though at that time the situation seemed extremely difficult, there is always some light at the end of the tunnel and that light in her life was the arrival of her unborn child. From that moment on and due to our respective circumstances, we became very good friends. During the following months we were partners at war, each one fighting our own difficult battle. From that day on, we were always together because unconsciously we were giving lots of support to one another. She would take me back and forth to the hospital as her companion when she visited her doctors during the pregnancy. Sandra's situation helped me to understand how everybody in life goes through difficult moments, but we all need to face them and try to resolve them in the best possible way. Because of the time that I spent with her, I learned that nobody has happiness guaranteed. By facing the whole world alone with her problem, she taught me a new meaning to the word "strength."

I was getting a lot of emotional support during the time that my mother was staying with us. She was helping me around the house with the children. I had a lot of friends constantly visiting me. It was during those six weeks that doubt and uncertainty seemed to overcome me. Every discomfort my body felt would terrify me since I imagined that the cancer was manifesting itself in another way or in some other place. Although I tried to avoid thinking about it, I kept asking myself if the doctors had removed every bad cell from my body. I couldn't avoid being pessimistic, thinking that maybe the stains that they had seen in my lungs and in my back just before my surgeries were dormant manifestations of cancer. Even though I tried not to think about this, I found myself going over it several times.

Those weeks of recovery were full of doubts, agony and suppressed emotions. I didn't want those around me to worry from seeing me suffering. It was a very difficult time during which I learned to treasure my moments of solitude.

During that time, my friend Raouf brought me as a gift an antique bell that I put next to my bed on my nightstand. I started using it every time I needed to call my children, my mother or Adela because they couldn't always hear me since my voice was so weak. The idea of using the bell was something that my children really liked. The moment I would ring the bell, they both would be by my bed to find out what I needed. It's funny how a simple detail such as this can motivate a child in such a special way. They would run to be at my side, feeling very important responding to their mother's call.

On the sixth weekend, Antonio talked to me about a surprise that he had prepared for me. He kept assuring me that I was going to enjoy it. He hadn't told me what it was, but he had talked about it with my mother. They had agreed that she would take me to the heliport on Saturday morning. Besides being a professional soccer player and actor, Antonio is a helicopter pilot. He had coordinated with his friend and instructor, Captain Elías, to take me to enjoy a helicopter ride through the skies of this beautiful city. When I found out about the surprise, I reacted with some incredulity. I don't know if I was afraid that it wasn't going to happen or of something else, but I was thrilled and very happy. We arrived at the heliport, which is located right near the port of Miami. It was a spectacular day in which the sun was shining brightly and reflecting intensely on the ocean. The almost cloudless sky seemed to be inviting us to come up. The helicopter was only a two-seater and didn't have side doors, making the adventure really intense because only the seat belt was keeping me from falling out. Before we took off, I felt a knot in my stomach. I was a little bit nervous, but the captain and Antonio kept cheering me up and they made me feel comfortable so that I could enjoy such a special ride. I was sitting in the co-pilot's seat. We finally took off just above the port's channel that led to the ocean. My heart was beating strongly. I was full of emotions in a special way. To tell the truth, I was a little bit nervous because I wasn't sure that physically my body was going to be able to withstand so much excitement.

We flew above the city and the shoreline for 45 minutes. I couldn't have asked for a better day to enjoy the view. We flew above the city's skyscrapers. From up there, I was able to appreciate the beautiful nature that makes this city extraordinary. Captain Elías really tried very hard to take me for an especially exciting ride. He achieved it. We flew above pristine beaches, little islands full of palm trees with incredible foliage, and the immensity of a sea that had an intense blue color on that day. Once up there I began to cry full of emotion and happiness because I felt that I was starting to live again. Those were tears of gratefulness, for I was truly fortunate to be able to enjoy life one more time. A feeling of well-being that I hadn't experienced in a long time was starting to take over my body. Being up there—amidst that special connection between nature and life—made me realize that I still had a long way to go, a lot of world to see, and much life to live. I felt a total identification with the universe. The feeling of being alive was overwhelming.

This special trip made me aware that life lasts only an instant. We can only take with us our soul and experiences, and what we enjoyed, went through and learned. Being up there, I was able to perceive the great contrasts that life has to offer. I became a poet for a moment and a philosopher for another, as I felt the paradox of life. I lived and day-dreamed, but above everything I felt alive once again—a feeling that for some time had been taken away from me. I appreciated the purity of nature, as I compared the blue of the ocean and the green of the trees with the concrete and glass of the skyscrapers. I perceived among the people on the beaches the excitement of those who enjoy nature, comparing it to the life of the bankers in the buildings of the city. I questioned the reason of my existence. And for the first time in a long while, I was thinking freely, I was feeling, I was living. I was able to compare my departure from life with the movement of the helicopter as it climbed nearer to the clouds. I realized that, even though they were waiting for me below, if I would have died, life would go on without me. Every time we flew close to the people below us I wanted to scream at them, "Look at me, I'm alive!" Although I didn't scream it out loud, I did scream it inside. I felt it. I lived it. That strong scream came from the deepest part of my heart and helped me to want to live, to hold on to life, and to give me determination, because I definitely wanted to continue to be alive.

It's curious how life's roads are formed, and how doors open and opportunities present themselves just at the right time. Since I had moved to Miami, I had always wanted to fly in a helicopter but hadn't done it. However, on that day, thanks to the kindness and generosity of two men that came upon my path, another dream was becoming a reality. It is amazing how such a simple detail as this could have had such a great impact in my recovery and motivation to live again. That gift from my very special friend gave a new perspective to my life. The time and effort of the Captain made it a reality. What an awesome way to feel alive again!

ADELA

I had been living in Miami for about a year when I hired a housekeeper by the name of Adela. Originally from Colombia, she was in the United States due to family issues at the time when my previous housekeeper had left me. When I first met her, I thought she was a rather elegant lady and I doubted that she really wanted to work in my house as a housekeeper. The salary that I could afford to pay her at that time wasn't as high as what other housekeepers were making in my same building. She was in need of a place where she could work and live, so it worked out well for both of us.

From the very beginning there was a good connection between her and my children. She was a grandmother herself and knew how to make children feel special without spoiling them, while at the same time keeping them well behaved. After some time I realized that she really liked us. As it's often the case when someone outside of the family lives with you, we started treating her like one of us.

At that time, Adela worked in my house for about a year until her visa expired and she had to go back to her country. We were rather sad with her departure because we grew to like her very much. When she left, she told me it was going to be temporary until she could apply for her visa to come back again.

A few weeks before she was to return to Colombia, she received a phone call from her daughter telling her that one of her sisters was very sick with stomach problems. She was very concerned, feeling helpless because of being away from home. Her sister was in and out of the hospital for a week until they finally called her with the bad news that she had cancer. Adela was torn up. She didn't want to leave my house without making sure that I found a trustworthy person to take over her responsibilities. At that time, I had just launched my new TV series and I really needed someone at home to help me with my children. Finding somebody suitable for the job took us about two or three weeks, delaying her departure longer than anticipated. I was feeling uneasy knowing that her sister was ill and she wouldn't go back home, but I think that deep inside she didn't really want to go back because she was afraid of her sister's true condition. She finally left one day. Unfortunately, her sister passed away just at the moment that her plane was landing in Bogota. She never got to say goodbye to her. I know that it had been very hard on her, especially since she didn't make it on time to say goodbye to her closest sister before the terminal disease took its toll.

On several occasions, Adela and I had talked about the possibility of her coming back to live with us when the lady that was replacing her would leave. That is one of the reasons why we kept in contact via telephone and Internet. My children asked about her constantly. We missed her a lot and liked getting news from her. I think that deep inside they could relate to her as the grandmother that they didn't have close to them and had shared so many special times of their childhood with them.

A few days after I had received my diagnosis, I sent her an e-mail giving her the bad news. Although she was so far away from us, she was always concerned about our health and well-being. At that time I wanted her to come back to accompany us through that Difficult Journey. I knew that I was going to feel better if she was in charge of my house because my children were going to be well taken care of and protected. Upon reading the news she called me, offering to work very hard to get her visa sooner. Trying to get a visa from Colombia is a matter of luck. It can take a couple of weeks or a couple of years. Although I still had the other lady in my house, the feeling was not the same. The first few days after receiving my diagnosis were very chaotic, but since I knew my mother and some of my brothers were going to be here, there was no hurry for Adela to come right away.

Just a few days before I had my first set of surgeries, the lady that was helping me at home informed me that she had to leave unexpectedly because her husband was ill. I didn't worry too much about her leaving because I knew that Adela was coming back and that my mother was going to be here in the meantime. I decided not to look for anybody else at that time. Although I knew that the surgeries were going to be hard, I was more afraid about the chemotherapy. I thought I would rather have her during the chemotherapy period because I was really going to need her then.

About a week after leaving the hospital following my first set of surgeries, we were finishing dinner when somebody knocked on my door. It was around 10 o'clock in the evening. My mother and I looked at each other, wondering who it might be at that time. Tommy opened the door and was surprised to see Adela right outside our door. She had come with a little suitcase, ready to start working that same evening. I was very happy to see her even though I was concerned because I had just found out how much money I owed to the hospital and I had an idea of how many bills were coming, which made me worry about not having enough money to pay her salary. I felt so sick that it took me only a minute to realize that due to my physical condition I really needed her with me. She had never called me to give me a specific date for her return, catching me a little off guard. But she explained to me that she had decided not to let me know that she was coming because she didn't want me to ask her to stay in Colombia a little bit longer because my mother was with me at home. She said she spent her days imagining how difficult my situation was at home, making her very worried being very far from us, so she just packed her bags, took a flight and came straight to us.

The first few days that she spent with us everything was good and relaxed. A couple of weeks later, however, I started to feel some friction between my mother and her. Since they were both pretty much the same age, I felt they were kind of competing to see who was the best cook or who would play better with my children. I kind of thought that something like that was going to happen but, to tell the truth, I had so many other concerns in my life that I tried to ignore their comments to each other, which sometimes made me feel uncomfortable. With Adela in charge of my house, all of the sudden my mother had too much free time on her hands. Besides taking my children to and from school, mother didn't have anything else to do. I started to sense that she was feeling uncomfortable. Whenever there was a day in which I felt more or less OK, I would ask Sandra to pick me up and take me for a ride, a visit to the office, or just to drive around. I began to feel that if I wasn't feeling sick or in pain and would leave the house for more than a couple of hours, my mother would think she could not justify her time with us and, perhaps, that she was wasting her time. I could understand that it wasn't easy for her because she had been with us for two and a half months. When you haven't lived together for 19 years, so much time living under the same roof is not easy to do, especially under those circumstances. Even though we have a cordial relationship that has gotten better with the years, she was always a lot closer to my sister than to me. Although my children are her oldest grandchildren, she had never spent more than a week's time with them. I am very grateful for the time that she stayed with us, even though I knew from the very beginning that she was battling internally between wanting to spend time with us and wanting to go back home to her own life. Spending so much time with a sick person is not easy. It is not easy whether you are the mother, the father, the son, the daughter, the niece, the uncle or the grandchild. Being with a sick person is simply not easy. It is necessary to understand that.

After talking to Adela and making sure that she wasn't going to leave us until I had finished my treatments, I decided to talk honestly with my mom regarding her stay with us. I started by telling her how grateful I was to her for taking time off from her work, friends and life to come help me during this difficult time. Then, I explained to her that sometimes I felt that she was making me feel bad unintentionally, because whenever I was able to leave home with my friends for some time she was in a bad mood whenever I came back. It is as if I was feeling that she needed to know that I was sick so she would feel better by being there. I tried to make her understand that due to my difficult situation I needed to take advantage of the few days in which I had some energy to try to do everyday things. I couldn't comprehend why she needed to feel that I had to be sick for her to feel all right. I suggested that she should go back home for awhile and asked her to come back and spend some time with us during my radiation therapy since I felt that we all needed a break and she would help me more by coming back after being away for sometime. She was very concerned about what my brothers were going to think of her if she went back home without me finishing my recovery. I had to make her understand that whatever they thought was irrelevant. As I usually say, it is very easy to give advice about what somebody else has to do, but it is very difficult to make the sacrifice and dedicate your own time for the well-being of somebody else.

After our brief conversation, I could see that she was really anxious to leave and get back to her life. After three days she got an airplane ticket and left. On the day of her departure, I was very sad to see her leave. She was totally excited about going to her home, her friends and her world. Although I understood her excitement, I would have liked it if she could have been able to feel more comfortable being with us. I guess that, in a selfish way, I was thrilled with having my mother by my side all along my Difficult Journey.

Once my mother left, Adela felt more relaxed and I think that from that moment on she decided to "adopt" me as her daughter. It was a strange feeling, but I felt some kind of relief right after I came home from dropping my mother off at the airport because, somehow, my house was again my home like it had been before my illness: my children, Adela and me.

The chemotherapy period was terrible, as I describe it in the chapter dedicated to that topic, but in this chapter I want to mention that Adela took extraordinary care of me during those months. She was truly outstanding. She kept an eye on me night and day. She paid attention to the most minimal details, such as making sure that I had my pitcher of water at my nightstand every night. She would open the windows of my apartment every time she cooked so that the smell wouldn't make me nauseous. She would wash my clothes and dishes separate from my children's to make sure I wouldn't get any germs. She cooked special meals to help me boost my immune system, even making fresh carrot juice for me every morning. She would check my phone calls and limit my friend's visits so I wouldn't get overly tired. The list of her special treatment is so long, I would need another chapter just to write about everything that she did for me during those few months. In a certain way, she assumed the roll of a mother. She did not leave my side until I had finished all of my treatments and gone on my first vacation with my children, almost a year later.

Although tension and minor problems were there on some days, as tends to happen in any relationship, Adela has been a marvelous human being with me. I will always be grateful to her for the care, dedication and love that she gave to me as well as my children. I know that it wasn't easy for her to leave her family behind to come to take care of my family. To her it was a sacrifice to leave her house, daughter and grandchildren, and that is something that only very special people are capable of doing. She is the one person who truly lived by my side during the whole process of this terrible illness, not being able to sleep many nights worried for my health and taking care of keeping my children happy, well-fed and busy. I believe that she has earned a seat in heaven for everything she did for us. Even though she was receiving a salary from me, she did her job with love, dedication and enthusiasm. The time she dedicated to us was priceless.

CHEMOTHERAPY

"My mommy is undergoing chemotherapy. This means that some small soldiers get inside her body, attack the cells and kill them. The bad thing is that they also kill the good cells that make the hair grow. So that's why my mommy has to wear hats, caps and bandanas. Poor mommy, she feels really sick."

— *Tommy*

During the two months following my surgeries I had to keep going constantly to see the doctors as well as to have a lot of tests done. For some reason, the functioning of my left kidney wasn't as they had anticipated, creating delays to the beginning of my chemotherapy. I was anxious to start the treatment because, although I knew that it was going to be difficult, I wanted to feel that I was doing everything possible to eradicate the illness and not continue to worry that it kept spreading in my body.

When finally the time came to choose a clinical oncologist to be in charge of my treatment, I talked to my friend Tito, the pathologist, and to Doctor D., my surgeon. They both suggested a female doctor that had her practice at the same hospital, with whom they had a good personal and professional relationship. They both agreed that she should be the doctor in charge of my chemotherapy. The idea of being treated by a female doctor was not very exciting to me at first because I had never been treated by a female physician in my life. I had no doubts whatsoever about the professional capability of female doctors, but throughout my life I have always had better relationships with men, in both personal and professional terms. After thinking about their recommendation for a few minutes, I decided to give it a try. I made an appointment to see her, knowing that I had nothing to lose by talking to her because they would help me find somebody else to take care of my treatment if I didn't feel comfortable with her.

The day of my first meeting with her, my mother went with me to her office, but stayed outside in the waiting room. She interviewed me in her office before performing a physical exam. I liked the fact that she took the time to get to know me a little bit before the first physical exam. We talked about my problem. She shared with me the statistics and gave me her recommendation as far as the treatment that she would like me to have. She gave me some options. We chatted and, after awhile, ended up looking at pictures of her daughters and family. I guess there was a common bond between us.

Due to the fact that my tight financial situation was always on my mind, I talked to her honestly about my lack of medical insurance and income. She looked at me a little bit surprised because, according to her, she would have never guessed that somebody with a television career could be in that position. After listening to me, she determined that due to my financial situation it would be better for me if I was able to receive chemotherapy right in the hospital as opposed to receiving it at her office since prices are higher in private practices. She also suggested that to save money I should get my weekly blood work done at the hospital. She also advised me on how to try to get some financial help from the hospital. Once again I felt very fortunate having found yet another doctor that was concerned about my personal situation because, as I mentioned before, after all the years of living in this country I had never been fortunate enough to deal with doctors with such compassion. She inspired a lot trust in me. I realized that, besides being very sensitive and caring, she was very professional. I decided right away that she would be the oncologist heading up my treatment.

During that first visit we worked on the schedule for my treatment. She talked to me about the side effects of that particular chemo and set a date in which I was to receive my first dose. She explained to me that my type of cancer was very aggressive and needed to be attacked aggressively. She told me that, as a result of the chemicals that were going to be used on me, I was going to lose my hair, gain weight and feel tired and nauseous. She talked to me about the progress of medicine during the last few years in respect to the minimization of the side effects. She gave me strength to face the treatment and continue with my fight against cancer. Out of everything she told me that day, what affected me the most was when she told me that my ovaries were going to be damaged and that, more than likely, I was never going to be able to have any more children. She told me that as if trying not to give it a lot of importance, knowing that I was without a partner at that time and I already had two healthy and beautiful children. She had no idea that one of my biggest dreams in life was to have at least another child at the age of 40. I don't know why, but I had always thought it was going to happen. It is so much so that my children knew that even if mommy wasn't married again, they would at least have another baby brother or sister at home. When I found out that such a special dream of mine wasn't going to come true due to the fact of this illness, I was very sad. Once again I experienced the helplessness and frustration that is felt while questioning the reason for having cancer.

Anyhow, I was fighting to stay alive at that time. I thought it was more important to be healthy for my two children than to have fantasies about having more children. I decided to accept any side effects that I had to face because it was going to be worth it to stay alive.

Among the recommendations the doctor gave me that day, she stressed the fact that I needed to have someone helping me with my children and with the household chores. She told me that I needed to learn to take advantage of the little energy that I was going to have during the months of treatment. She also suggested repeatedly that I needed to go out and shop for a wig and scarves to try to cover up my baldness. It seemed to me at that time that she was more concerned than I about my hair loss.

Before concluding the visit, a specialized nurse came to check my veins, making sure that they were strong enough to receive chemotherapy. Unfortunately, she didn't think they were, so the doctor explained to me that it was going to be necessary to install what is called a distribution port into my body. A distribution port is a small disc made out of metal or plastic that is surgically inserted under the skin and that has a catheter that travels from the chest to the heart. It is installed right in the superior vein, where the chemicals are pumped into the body. This port is installed and removed by a doctor who is specialized in this procedure at the hospital, requiring a hospital stay and anesthesia. While they were talking and giving me all of the explanations for their decision for me to have it, I could only imagine the cash register ringing up the costs in my mind, knowing that once again I needed to be in the hospital. I insisted on knowing if there was a way to avoid it, not only because of the money but also since the only place on my body that didn't have any scars at that time was my upper chest, which was where they needed to install the device. I tried as hard as I could, but wasn't able, to convince them that my veins were good enough. Right then, they set up a date for me to go into the hospital to have this procedure done. I was disappointed because, besides being uncomfortable, I was adding another scar to my body.

Without a doubt the most difficult time of my life has been the time that I underwent chemotherapy. The sensations that I went through during those months were extremely difficult, physically and emotionally. It is a period of time that to this day is difficult to talk or write about. Although mentally I thought I was prepared to start the treatment, actually going through it was extremely difficult.

The day of my first session, Antonio came to pick me up and take me to the hospital. That morning I had a lot of mixed feelings. I was afraid, worried, anguished and, of course, fearful because I didn't know what to expect. Although I had read a lot about chemotherapy and its possible side effects, I can honestly tell you that I did not read anywhere what I felt and experienced at that time. I don't know if it is that I am a very sensitive person or if my body reacted in a different way, but the chemotherapy period has been the most difficult of my entire life. I don't think I was prepared to handle it.

When we got to the room in which I was going to be receiving the treatment, I noticed three people receiving their own treatment. Everybody was quiet and they were lying down in beds with the bottles of chemicals connected to them. Two older men and a very old lady who was accompanied by her daughter were there. Once again I felt this strange sensation of being too young to be facing this. I didn't have much time to think about it because the nurse, Sheila, came to introduce herself and began talking to me. She wanted to know how I felt. She explained to me what I needed to expect when I left the hospital after having received the chemicals. She prepared the needles, uncovered my chest, found the distribution port, cleaned the area, and got me ready. Antonio left the room to go to the cafeteria, where he was meeting a friend whom he hadn't seen for a long time. I was frightened and would have liked for him to stay with me, but I didn't tell him anything. I tried to be brave. Although I was about to cry, I didn't. Sheila sat right in front of me and began explaining what she was doing step by step. It seemed to me that she was speaking in a strange language because I didn't understand half of what she was saying. She realized how nervous and scared I was. She called a counselor to talk to me and calm me down. I felt better after talking to her and telling her my fears, and finding the answers to some of my questions. A few minutes later, I began to feel how the chemicals were entering my body and started to have a metal sensation on my palate. I felt as if I had sniffed water up my nose. I began to take deep breaths and tried to start meditating to find some peace within myself. I kept repeating to myself in silence, "Everything is going to be all right. Everything is going to be all right." Although I knew that those chemicals were helping me to kill the bad cells, I was still very afraid, worried and concerned.

Without any major problems, the session ended two hours later after finally receiving my first dose. Feeling uncomfortable and uneasy, I was very anxious to leave the hospital and go home. Antonio and his girlfriend showed up to pick me up. I was feeling sick and the last thing I wanted was to be socializing. I thought it was rather imprudent of him to pick me up with her along, but I tried to show a good face and be courteous while we walked to the car. I got into my car and all I wanted to do was leave the hospital right away, but he took a while longer walking her to her car. Without them seeing me, I began to cry while I was waiting for him. On the way home I was feeling sick. I was very fragile emotionally. The thing that I wanted the most at that time was to feel safe. Unfortunately, nobody from my family had been able to be with me, even though I had called them and asked if they could. I had called my sister and two of my brothers the previous week asking them if they could arrange to be with me. On that difficult and lonely day, the reasons that the three of them had given me for not being with me kept coming to my mind, making me feel worse. My sister told me she had to go to a party that she could not miss. My two brothers told me that they had to work. I felt so alone in the middle of this terrible storm. I was very frightened. Unfortunately, I realized that, even though my life had changed so drastically and suddenly, everybody else was living his or her lives without realizing the tremendous anguish that I was feeling. At that time I learned to value the time dedicated to me by those who truly loved me.

Since the day of my first session was a Friday, I had asked Tom to take the children to his house over the weekend because I didn't want them to see me coming back from the hospital. After all it was only my first dose and I didn't know how I was going to react. My mother was in Texas taking care of some personal business and, although Adela was with me at home, I had asked Antonio to spend the night with me because I needed to feel that I was special to somebody. I didn't want to be alone.

While driving home, Antonio told me that he had just made plans to have dinner with his friend and asked me if I would mind if she could come to my place for a drink. Any other day I wouldn't have minded, but under those circumstances I thought it was totally inappropriate. I was going through one of the most difficult situations in my life and my best friend was thinking about going out on a date with someone that he hadn't seen in months and could see on any given day. I was very sad because I was feeling abandoned not only by my family but also by him, whom I practically consider my brother. We argued a little bit about it, but I didn't have the strength or desire to fight. I believe that he never quite understood what I was going through at that time. All I wanted was to know that I was special to somebody. I wanted to feel that somebody who loved me was taking care of me and that what was happening to me was important to somebody. I needed to know that at least someone was concerned about my health. The last thing that I wanted that day was the company of strangers. I needed to feel special and just wanted to rest.

We arrived at my house. Adela opened the door, hugged me, and took me to my bedroom. I didn't want to take any calls because I needed to be alone in my room. Antonio left, but the bad feelings stayed with me. I lay down on top of my bed with the same clothes that I was wearing. Shortly after, I started vomiting. My house felt strange. It was very empty without my children. I was emotionally devastated.

Antonio came back that night to see how I was feeling. He walked into my room, sat on the bed next to me, took out my laptop and started checking his e-mail. Once he finished, he left the room. A little later I heard the TV in the living room and shortly after he was singing on my terrace outside. I would have liked for him to stay next to me, just keeping me company. I was feeling terribly alone. I guess that, to him, being in my house was tantamount to keeping me company. It's hard for me to explain how on that particular night I felt totally alone and outside of myself. I could not sleep. I kept throwing up constantly. Around three in the morning, between crying and vomiting, I picked up the phone and called my friend Cristina, who lives in Los Angeles. As soon as she answered the phone,

I started crying for the longest time. I was feeling a lot of sadness and needed to talk to someone. A lot of pressure had built up over so many months, surgeries, and changes in my life. That night, I couldn't take it anymore. I think that particular night was the most difficult of all during the whole process of my illness because I realized at last how hard it is to face such a big disease without the company of your family. Even today, I remember that night as the loneliest night of my life.

The nausea was terrible, even though I had taken the pills that the doctor gave me. I couldn't keep from throwing up again about every half-hour. I had nothing left in my stomach, so I was simply throwing up bile. After several hours of constant vomiting, I started feeling weak and getting very frustrated because I couldn't stop throwing up. I wanted to remain calm, but the slightest movement made me throw up again. Those were three intensely difficult days that I spent going back and forth from my bed to my bathroom.

On the second day, I started feeling very tired. It was a strange feeling. I felt exhausted as if I had exercised a lot. I didn't have any more strength in my body. I remember that I would stay totally still in my bed, staring at the ceiling and thinking that I didn't even have the strength to move my hand to reach for the TV remote control. I couldn't even bear the thought of reading a book because the mere thought of the book's weight was tiring. It is difficult to explain how tired I was.

On that second day, my mother came to Miami to spend a few days with me, but she went back to Mexico for good before I had my second dose.

The third day after the chemotherapy was the worst. I had spent three days vomiting constantly, growing more tired and weak, and started to get depressed. I began to analyze how difficult my situation was and felt really down. I literally did not stop crying for even a moment during those days. On that third day and one day after each chemo session, I felt so exhausted physically and emotionally that I asked myself if the fight was worth it. I honestly thought about loosing the battle and letting myself die. It seems incredible. I am generally a very positive woman. I consider myself a fighter and a persevering person, but on that third day and for at least one day after each session, I felt that life was escaping from my hands and that I wasn't capable to continue fighting to try to live. My only rays of hope on those days were my children. Their company, words, tenderness and, especially, their unconditional love was what gave me the strength I needed not to allow myself to be defeated. Those little people, those special little people, made me hang on to life.

Chemotherapy in itself is a combination of chemicals designed to kill cancerous cells. One of the bad things about the treatment is that it attacks all cells that multiply rapidly in the same manner, regardless if they are cancerous or not, which is why you lose your hair. Chemotherapy can affect the bone marrow by limiting the amount of white cells that it can produce, therefore making the patient more susceptible to any germs or diseases. That is the reason why the level of activities allowed to be taken on during treatment is very limited. While on treatment, public places should be avoided, as should contact with ill people and children who have received vaccinations. Hands should be washed constantly. Personal items should not be shared with anybody. In short, extreme measures should be taken in order to avoid being exposed to germs or viruses, even though, generally speaking, the good cells start to reproduce again after chemotherapy is finished. While undergoing chemo, it is necessary to have a blood count on a regular basis. Although it may seem that the blood work is the least dramatic part of the process, having had to go to the hospital once or twice a week to have my blood checked wasn't exactly easy. Several times, new young nurses without much experience with needles had to perform the job. On several occasions, they had to stick me more than once to be able to get the sample. If my blood count was lower than acceptable, my trips to the hospital had to be four or five times a week. Every single one of those tests was performed at the hospital in the same room in which the chemotherapy was administered to me. Unconsciously, my mind created a connection with the room that made me feel apprehensive as soon as I walked in. On one occasion, my blood count was so low that it became necessary for me to receive a blood transfusion.

During the five months that I received chemotherapy, every single aspect of my life was being affected by the severity of the treatments. As I have written before, due to the aggressiveness of my cancer, the plan of attack was just as aggressive. Nevertheless, when the doctors warned me before the chemo about the severity of the treatment, they fell short in communicating its intensity. Many were the days that I asked myself what would kill me first, the cancer or the chemotherapy. The queasiness and the nausea, vomiting, overexhaustion, sleepiness, fatigue, severe pain in my legs, and depression from seeing myself physically in bad shape, tired, swollen, bloated and pale every single day, made it even harder. In short, I felt that the chemotherapy was killing me before bringing me back to life.

My chemotherapy cycle consisted of one dose every three weeks. Usually, the first week was very cloudy, mentally speaking, because my days were spent vomiting, trying to sleep, trying to get up to vomit some more, and trying to sleep again. On the second week, the nausea diminished a little bit, but the exhaustion and the pains in my legs grew stronger. The chemotherapy damaged the muscles in my legs, so it began to be very difficult for me to stand up and even walk. I was very fortunate to have my legs massaged by my friend, Isabel. Those massages helped the pain to be less intense, especially during the first few days after each dose. I took advantage of the third week, which was when I was starting to come to life again and needed to be recovering my strength before being "tortured" again, to get away with my children to Islamorada. Islamorada, easily accessible by car, is located just south of Miami in the Florida Keys. Being there represented a direct contact with the greatness of nature. I had discovered a small hotel just at the water's edge. It wasn't anything elegant or fancy, but it was very homey. Each room had its own kitchen and bathroom, two double beds, and big terraces. In this place, my children spent their days picking up shells from the sand, swimming in the clear waters, playing basketball and tennis, fishing from the pier, and enjoying the warm translucent water of the ocean. In the meantime, I would spend my days lying down on a lounge chair simply staring at the immensity of the ocean, thinking, reflecting about life, and being grateful for the lessons I was learning. During these trips I had the opportunity to establish a very strong spiritual connection between myself, the Supreme Being and nature. I was able to discover several faces of myself that I didn't know until that time. I had time to reflect and try to understand the different lessons that I was learning while living with cancer. I felt very privileged to be able to spend so much time on this island during my therapy. The direct contact with the greatness of creation enriched my soul and gave me strength to continue during that Difficult Journey.

During the period of recovery from my surgeries and just before the beginning of my first chemotherapy, I went to a luncheon at my friend Aida's house. She was throwing a housewarming party. Although I didn't feel like going, my mother insisted that it would be good for me to go as a distraction and to break the monotony. Aida is a very positive and hardworking businesswoman whom I admire very much. She usually has very interesting guests in her house. During that luncheon I met Lilia, a beautiful and elegant lady who became another one of my angels for many months.

From the moment we met, we found a lot of things in common with each other. After talking for a little bit, we started developing a very close bond. She is a woman who, besides being beautiful, is a spiritual and very enlightened human being who has given the world, through her books and speeches, a large amount of information and knowledge on the esoteric plane.

She took me under her wing from the very beginning of our relationship and was always concerned about my health, progress and treatment. The most beautiful gift that she gave me during my treatment was her time, spending hours keeping me company in my house. She went to most of my chemotherapy sessions to help me meditate while I was receiving the chemicals. Once the nurse had started the treatment, Lilia and I would close our eyes. She would then hold my hand and help me visualize the liquids that I was receiving as carriers of good health that were helping me to battle the mistake that was inside my body. She taught me to receive the treatment with love and bless it for being and integral part of my curative process. During those sessions, her voice would guide me through a road of peace and harmony. A couple of times I got so relaxed that

I felt that the cleansing of the cells was also the cleansing of my soul.

Due to the fact that the room in which my chemo was administered to me was not a private suite, we had to whisper while meditating in order not to bother the other people. From my second session, I was fortunate to have been accompanied by more than one person close to me while I was receiving treatment. Besides Lilia, Juan was by my side during those days and my father and brother, Ricardo, would take turns visiting me. However, once the moment of the needles arrived, the guys would always find an excuse to go down to the cafeteria to pass the time until my treatment was finished. I sort of understand it because, even though males are supposed to be the stronger sex, I think that inside hospitals they become the weaker sex.

Through meditations with Lilia I learned to communicate with my body and cells—even the tiniest of them—asking and ordering them to be cured. I began to understand the importance of meditation in order to achieve harmony inside our bodies. I learned a lot about the protection, presence and importance of our guardian angels.

During the whole process of recovery, I placed my life in the hands of my guardian angels, asking them for guidance and protection. The most shocking thing of it all is that the results of their protection and generosity have truly been tangible. I have always known that I am a very fortunate person who walks in this world under the protection of a very special angel. Through this illness, I have realized that there is a full team of angels protecting and taking care of me from the world beyond.

I have always considered myself to be a very spiritual person who bases her life more on the intangible than on the tangible. Because of this illness, I feel that I have gotten very close to the Supreme Being and the greatness and magnitude of His kindness.

I have crossed paths with many good and generous people during the course of my life. Throughout my process of recovery, I have received innumerable blessings along the way. I have discovered that the mind plays a very important role in the health of human beings because we are capable of attracting or pushing away illnesses with our thoughts. Although scientifically it's very hard to prove this concept, I choose to believe it is true. I'm beginning to see the results of my findings now that I've come out of my Difficult Journey.

From my very personal point of view, I think that a good relationship between body and mind is the essence of finding a cure for any kind of illness. During this process I came to the conclusion that it's the mind that unconsciously brings up the illness. This is a strong and hard statement to accept, especially if we do not like to bring harm to others or ourselves. I am convinced that the stress we put ourselves through, the fast-paced lifestyle, the pressures of society, the worries and the lack of a well-balanced diet are some of the factors that contribute to an imbalance between our bodies and our soul and to a manifestation of illnesses. It seems to me that the feelings of anger, rage, bad feelings, sadness, hurt, and all of the negative energies that are not channeled correctly are equally important in contributing to physical damage.

Even though there is no medical way to prove the relationship between body and soul, a positive attitude towards life is absolutely indispensable to combat and overcome any type of illness. Life has several intangibles that do not materialize but do exist, and we simply know and accept them. Love, for example, is a sentiment that we simply feel and fills us with happiness, joy and satisfaction. I believe that, in the same way, a cure can manifest itself once we are able to harmonize our own life. I believe that true happiness can be reflected in our bodies once we achieve true happiness in our souls.

I know there will be those who believe in this approach to life and those who won't. In my own case, I believe it helped me. I am the kind of person who tends to do in life what I believe is good for myself, even if it is not necessarily the most conventional approach.

During the months of chemotherapy, all of my activities were severely reduced because my energy level was very low. I had to learn to limit the number of things that I could do each day. I wanted to maximize the little strength I had to be able to spend some time talking to my children when they came home from school or from their summer camp. For the first time in many years, I learned to say no when I didn't feel like doing something.

Another stroke of luck along the way was finding the generosity of my friend Raúl. He was the director of the tennis summer camp that my children attended. Besides giving them a full scholarship for the summer, he would personally pick them up and bring them back home every single day. To my children, that summer was very special because, in a certain way, they were known at the camp as the director's special friends. That motivated them to become even greater players since they wanted Raúl and me to be very proud of them.

Being a very social person, one of the hardest things for me to do was learning to stop answering the phone calls from all my friends and asking them to limit their visits if I wasn't feeling strong enough to keep up a conversation. I have never been the kind of person who tells a friend to leave my house, but under those circumstances I felt an obligation to myself to limit the amount of time that I spend with somebody besides my children. I am very fortunate to have been surrounded by a lot of wonderful and unselfish people, which is what really counts in life because unconditional love enriches our souls and our lives.

Reflecting on the chemotherapy period, I think it is important to emphasize that the care and love that can be instilled in the self indispensable in order to achieve a quick recovery. During that time, it became very important for me to reflect, to get close to my inner self and to learn to heal my soul. Once I started to heal myself emotionally, my body started to heal itself physically.

It is important to stress that during that period of time it was necessary to detach myself from so many mundane, trivial and unimportant matters that could easily absorb what little energy I had left.

I believe it's important for those who spend time around a sick person to understand that the sick need to have their own time and space, and that doesn't mean that they do not appreciate the company, good intentions and love of others. In my particular case, I needed many days to be totally alone so as not to be drained of my energy.

I do not tire of saying that chemotherapy is a very difficult process. That's just the way it is. Even though several people told me about the great advances in this type of treatment over the last 20 years, I can't even imagine how somebody could have felt any worse than I did. Chemotherapy was brutal. Even today I doubt that I would put myself through it one more time if I ever have cancer again. Besides being physically excruciating, chemotherapy is mentally devastating. Not only did I feel sick, but I was also very tired, sensitive, irritable, susceptible, totally bald, without either eyebrows or eyelashes and bloated. As if the harshness of the treatments weren't enough, slowly but surely I started feeling my clothes tighter. When the treatments finally ended, I was 14 pounds heavier.

Besides having to go through all the torture, at the end of the treatment I was fat and bald, even though I knew that this was only temporary, but while I was living it, it was my reality and a very difficult one to accept.

IT'S ONLY HAIR

"When my mommy had long hair, she looked better. When she had short hair, she looked bad. When she had long hair in the pictures, she was always smiling and happy, but when she had short hair in the pictures, she looked sad. Now that she doesn't have any hair in the pictures, she looks tired and sick."

—*Izzy*

From the first visit to the oncologist and her explanation of the chemotherapy treatment, what I had suspected was confirmed: I was going to lose my hair due to the use of a particular drug. At that time, my concern was about fighting for my life, so the thought of losing my hair didn't really worry me too much, or at least I thought. I always knew that I had been privileged because I was born with well-defined facial features, but despite of this I have never been a vain person. I thought the hair would grow again and I would take advantage of it falling out to have a short and kind of half-crazy hairstyle that I always wanted to have, but didn't have the guts to do before.

Since I had read a lot about cancer and its treatments from the moment I started my Difficult Journey, I decided to cut my hair short bit by bit so that my children would get used to my changes. When I discovered the tumor, my hair was almost down to my waist so I decided to have it cut just above shoulder length. When I visited my hairdresser, she was very surprised when I asked her to cut my hair shorter since she used to enjoy giving me wild hairstyles every time that I went to social functions. She tried to convince me not to cut my hair short yet. I explained to her my situation, knowing she would eventually be the one who would shave my hair off. She wished me luck and gave me a very pretty haircut that made me look and feel younger.

That very same day when I picked up my children from school, they both told me how much they liked my haircut. Izzy asked me to take her to my hairdresser to have her hair cut just like mine. That gesture was enormously moving to me because I knew that what she wanted for a long time was to have her hair very long. She used to spend hours brushing her hair, trying to make it grow faster. I knew that she was showing her support by asking me to cut her hair just like mine. We are proud that people tell us how much she and I look alike. I held her tightly. The following day, I took Izzy with me to my hairdresser.

After the first week of chemotherapy I started to notice how I was losing my hair. It wasn't anything dramatic, but a few hairs would fall while combing or taking a shower. One day, my mother came home with a bag full of scarves in anticipation of when I would need to cover my head. I decided to start wearing them right away to get used to it and also because bandanas were in fashion at that time.

Two weeks after my first dose, I woke up with a strange kind of headache. It was as if my hair roots were hurting me, kind of like when you change the direction in which you comb your hair. As soon as I touched my head to ease the pain, clumps of hair would fall out. That morning I called the children into my room and asked them to pull at my hair, take the big lumps in their hands and throw them into the trash can. They were feeling shocked and afraid. At that moment I knew that the time of becoming bald was almost there.

A couple of days later, I took my shower in the morning before going to the office. When I dried my hair and started combing it, I felt a weird sensation. Looking at myself in the mirror, I saw two huge white spots the size of a fist on top of my head, where the skin was totally white. I couldn't believe that I had lost a lot of hair all of a sudden and had bald spots in my head. I sat right in front of my mirror and I started crying. I cried silently because I didn't want my mother, Adela or my children to hear me. Even though I knew it was coming, it was difficult to see myself bald. After a few minutes of anguish, I took a deep breath and exited my room wearing my pink bandana. I called Sandra and asked her to come and pick me up to take me to the hair salon because the time had come to have my head shaved. On my way there I told her what had happened in the bathroom but she really didn't believe me. I guess she thought I was exaggerating.

As soon as we got to the salon, my hairdresser came over and said hello to us. Seeing some hair under my bandana, she thought that I was rushing things and started telling me about one of her friends from Paris that went through chemotherapy but never really lost her hair. I know she was trying to cheer me up and was grateful for her good intentions. When I removed my bandana from my head, she and Sandra stared at me, looked at each other, and understood immediately that I needed to shave the rest of it. "It's only hair. It will come back again," they kept telling me. That was the first time that I heard the phrase that would follow me during the next eight months of my life: "Its only hair." Hair. That's right! Only hair. Hair that will eventually grow back. Hair that, at that particularly moment, was the physical representation of the illness that I was trying to fight. My bald head meant "I have cancer."

It probably seems silly to dedicate a whole chapter of my book to my lack of hair, but lack of hair was an integral part of my life for several months. The first few days as a bald woman were difficult. They were difficult because I wasn't used to looking at myself in the morning and seeing a bald person. They were difficult because I wasn't used to having to cover my head before leaving the house. They were difficult for my children because they had never seen mommy bald. They were difficult for my friends because we all knew that it was "only hair." During that period of time, the lack of hair was the affirmation that cancer existed. Although the hair fell off due to the chemicals they were giving me, the lack of hair was a constant reminder that I had that terrible illness.

Slowly but surely, I was becoming braver. I started to show my baldhead in public, but it wasn't easy. Even though in my house it was "al natural" from the beginning, it was difficult to start seeing my friends with my new appearance. Many times the expression on people's faces tells you more than a lot of words. Although "it was only hair," many times people were feeling uncomfortable by just looking at me. They didn't know how to react or what to say. Some people tried to pretend that looking at me bald didn't bother them, but I know it did because they wouldn't look at me directly. Some other people would tell me that I looked good, but I knew that they were saying it out of compassion because I also had mirrors during this whole process. Although in the beginning "it was only hair," a few weeks later I also lost my eyebrows and my eyelashes. Antonio began calling me "baldy" and he enjoyed kissing my bald head. One of my girlfriends decided not to see me again until I had hair because it was too hard on her. My daughter, Izzy, liked caressing and massaging my bald head. She kept telling me that I looked like an extraterrestrial. My son, Tommy, decided not to touch my head because he thought it felt weird.

My new hobby became searching for and buying bandanas of all colors to match everything I would wear. The summer months in Miami are particularly hot. Although many times I just felt like walking out without covering my head, I didn't always have the guts to do it. I now realize that the simple act of walking bald in front of people is also part of the emotional process that goes along with the healing.

On a day that I wasn't feeling too bad, I made the huge effort of taking my children to the shopping mall because Tommy wanted to get a new pair of tennis shoes. While we were walking, I started feeling sick and had to sit down on a bench for a moment. I had the feeling that I was going to faint because I started suffocating. My first reaction was to remove my bandana from my head to cool myself off. As I was doing that, I noticed a mature looking woman staring at me in such a way that made me feel uncomfortable. I tried to ignore it and concentrated on calming myself down because I was alone with the kids. My children were concerned but were trying to cheer me up. A few minutes later, that same lady got together with a group of friends. My children and I noticed that they kept looking at me and were talking to each other. For some reason that woman wouldn't stop looking at us, making us feel uncomfortable. Shortly after, they walked next to us. Since she hadn't stopped staring, Tommy looked at and told her, "My mommy has cancer and she's not feeling well, so please stop staring." I was totally surprised at his reaction. From the very beginning of my illness, Tommy was very protective of me.

That incident was just one of the negative reactions that I encountered, but I can talk about many other positive ones. One that comes to mind was when my friend Raúl invited me for lunch. Raúl was the director of the tennis camp that my children were going to during the summer. I hadn't seen him in a few months and wasn't really very excited about having lunch at a nice restaurant looking like I did. He insisted so much on picking me up to take me for lunch that I had no choice but to accept. I met him in the front of my building. After hugging me, he told me that he had prepared a surprise for me. I looked at him as if in doubt. He removed his cap and what a surprise! He had shaved his head just to look like me. I thought that what he did was awesome!

One day I finally decided to go looking for a wig. Juan insisted on taking me to buy it since he claims to know what looks good on me and what doesn't. Besides being my friend, he was the producer of my TV show. Since we started working together, he somehow took it upon himself to always try to make me look better. He would always tell me which clothes looked nice on me and which didn't, which colors I should wear and which I shouldn't, so I let him continue with his fantasy of being my "image coordinator." To tell the truth, I wasn't that sure I wanted to buy a wig because I didn't even think that I was going to wear it, but it seemed interesting to experiment with a "new look".

We went to the wig shop that I was referred to by another chemotherapy patient I had met at the hospital. She knew of this place through her doctor. It was a place that specialized in supplying wigs to cancer patients. The gentleman who served me was very friendly and helped me to try on several different wigs before deciding which one to purchase. I opted to get one with very short hair and a color similar to my own hair color, but with a totally different style than I ever had. It was a very short hairstyle with spiky hair on the front. I chose that one because I wanted something totally different than what I was used to. Perhaps I was looking for something that would help me start living a new reality, helping me to forget what I was really going through. I don't know. Looking back at it, I think that the purchase of the wig was totally absurd and I didn't give it much use. I don't think I wore it more than a half dozen times. I only wore it to a couple of business meetings and other appointments with clients who didn't know about my situation. I didn't want to explain it the situation to them but, in reality, I wasn't used to wearing a wig and felt totally strange wearing one because I kept worrying that if I moved my head sharply it would fall off and people would laugh at me. On those few days that I wore it, Juan kept fixing it every 10 minutes. He constantly repeated to me how good I looked with it, giving me some confidence because Juan is totally upfront in that respect. Anyhow, I would have preferred not to wear it because I could never get used to it.

Losing hair during chemo is like a give and take. You first lose it little by little. Then it grows a little bit. Then big chunks come out. Then it starts growing again until one day you lose it all. It begins to grow again until the next dose when the process starts all over once more. Trying to make light of the situation, I decided to let some of my friends shave my head. That was a big event in my house. My children loved putting the shaving cream on my head before my friends would shave me.

Talking about baldness is strange. Under normal circumstances people don't pay so much attention to losing their hair. I have a lot of friends who have lost most of their hair and they have decided to shave their heads. I like how they look. Some of them look very handsome, but their situation is different. To them, becoming bald has been a natural process that has taken place gradually. It didn't happen overnight. They grow to accept it and see it as something normal. My case wasn't like that, because losing my hair overnight wasn't just about vanity. It was the constant reminder that I had cancer. Having no hair was definitely a very difficult stage of my Difficult Journey.

BEING A WOMAN

"My mommy doesn't have any hair. She looks like an extraterrestrial. She looks pretty, but like a pretty extraterrestrial. But she scares me anyway."

—*Izzy*

"When I see her scars, I feel bad. I don't like looking at them because I feel weird and I worry about her."

—*Tommy*

When I discovered I had cancer, I was living what I considered a normal lifestyle as far as what is normal for a contemporary single woman. I had divorced my second husband and father of my children three years before and moved to Miami with the hopes and dreams of establishing a business that would allow me to live comfortably while building the foundation for my children's future.

The intimate side of my life was what I considered good under my circumstances. When I first got married I was 21 years of age. I still don't understand why I did it since I was never in love with my first husband. Being very young and innocent, I needed an excuse to get out of my parent's house. I was a virgin until my honeymoon. Unfortunately, on our second night together, my problems with him started when he was arrested in a nightclub in Acapulco, but that's a story for another book. I grew up under a very strict education, not only at home but also at school. I attended the same all-girl Catholic school from the age of 5 until 18. Sex was something that we never talked about at home and rarely mentioned at school. Getting used to an active sex life has been something that has taken some time. I got divorced the first time before our second anniversary. Due to family pressure, I requested and received a church annulment.

In my continued search for happiness, I remarried four years later. Although I had two children with my second husband, our intimate life was almost nonexistent, creating one of our biggest problems.

Starting to date people my age after not having a lot of experience has been an adventure in itself. My dates have ranged from the most innocent, such as simply going for a coffee, to the most extravagant of evenings. I have dated a variety of men who have taken me out to dinners, movies and the like. I have had my share of happy times, sad times, excited times, and a couple of relationships that went nowhere.

When I found out I had cancer, I was going through a period of "emotional healing." A few months prior to my diagnosis, I thought I had fallen in love with someone that I even considered "the man of my life." I liked him physically and emotionally. I enjoyed his company and thought he was very intelligent, even though he gave me mixed signals from the very beginning. With time I realized that, although I loved him, that kind of love was not the love of a partner that I have sought for so long, but a certain kind of special love. We both loved each other very much, but we both carried a lot of baggage and had different expectations of life. When the breaking off of that relationship happened, it hit me very hard because, although I always considered it an emotional affair more than a physical one, we had invested a lot of time in it.

To try to forget him, I started to go out more, to meet more people and to accept more invitations. Being an attractive and sociable woman has opened a lot of doors, even in such a superficial society as the one I encountered in certain circles. At the risk of sounding immodest, I luckily have never lacked invitations from handsome men. The self-confidence and -trust that I was able to acquire during the two years that I had lived in Miami were being severely tested with this illness.

Surgeries, convalescence, recovery, chemotherapy, setbacks and radiation had me tired, a little bit depressed, and without any interest in leaving my house. Socializing during this period of time was totally out of the question. From being a very active and happy person, I became a rather insecure woman who sought refuge inside the comfort and security of her own house. I believe I was a little bit depressed because I was able to find excuses not to go out even on days when I was physically able to do so. At times it was as if I was afraid to face the world or see somebody that I had known and hadn't seen in a while because I didn't want to give explanations or talk about my illness anymore.

When I first had surgery, I couldn't even move. Recovery was painful and difficult. To remove the breast tumor, they cut into the right breast. To remove the lymph nodes, they went in under my armpit. And to remove the kidney tumor, they opened my abdomen just under my belly button with an incision that resembles the shape of a wave and extends to the rear of my left side. This last procedure required 56 stitches and was very tough physically.

During several weeks I was very happy just seeing my friends and family, whether at the hospital or at home. Starting to move again was difficult, so I adopted a routine. I would get up in the morning, sit next to my children while they had breakfast, and say goodbye to them when they went to school. Then I would go back to bed. An hour or so later, I would get up, take a shower, and dress in some of my pajamas, so I would look fresh and clean for my guests. Anticipating that I was going to be bedridden for a while, I went shopping to buy a lot of pajamas before going to the hospital. I figured that, if I was going to be sick and looking pale and ill, at least I should be wearing bright colored pajamas that would cheer me up. The necklaces that my children made and brought to the hospital for me became my lucky charms. I never took them off during the first three months after my surgery. During those months I read a lot of books, slept and rested a lot, and spent several hours a day just sitting on my balcony enjoying the beautiful view that I had of the city and the bay.

My only outings during the first two months were strictly to go to the doctor's office because the car ride made me dizzy. I had the good fortune of never feeling lonely since for a time my mother was with me, my sister and some of my brothers came to visit, and I always enjoyed the company of my friends, some of whom became my spiritual family. But even though I was feeling great love from the people around me, the happy, sure-of-herself and strong woman I was before cancer was slowly becoming an insecure, fragile and somehow reserved person, and I didn't understand why. I used to love parties, get-togethers and social events, yet suddenly I started to feel a certain fear of going out. Although the doctors had told me that I could go out, I didn't feel capable of doing so. Something inside me was preventing me from being Mayte. Looking at it in retrospect, I think that doubt towards my unknown future led me into depression, turning me into an insecure person.

The chemotherapy months were very difficult as a woman. As I wrote in another chapter, the loss of hair, although temporary, hits the female vanity in a very hard way. My self-esteem that had become strong during my couple of years in Miami was once again almost non-existent. From the time that I began my fight against cancer, I had gained 14 pounds, my clothes were tighter and, besides losing all of the hair from my head, my eyebrows and my eyelashes, I also lost my pubic hair. Looking at myself in the mirror, all I could see was a reflection of my illness and a constant reminder of the cancer. Although I would try to fix myself up everyday to look as good as possible, I felt uncomfortable with myself. A thousand times I would ask myself if I would ever again feel attractive as a woman.

Well, the day arrived and it came to me in the most unexpected way and with the least imagined person. Just a week after receiving my last dose of chemotherapy, Javier called me. He had been living in New York and was letting me know that he was going to be in Miami for a few days for work purposes. We had always kept in touch during the period of my illness, either by phone or by e-mail. He told me he was really looking forward to seeing me. We have been friends since childhood when we both lived in Mexico City. Although we were always attracted to each other, we never expressed this attraction since we were always involved with other people. Distance never got in the way of our friendship. Even though we lived in different cities, we always kept in touch. Our relationship throughout time can be summed up like that of two souls that meet each other sporadically but are always together sharing a spiritual love that transcends physical feelings because, even though it does not materialize, it can always be felt and is known to be there.

The first time we saw each other on this trip was when I went to the launching of his new album. His record label was promoting his new material by offering a cocktail party to which our industry's most influential people would be attending. Being aware of his guest list, I knew that going to the launch would be a great test for me. Besides seeing him, I would be surrounded by my peers, some of whom I hadn't seen for months. I decided to go. I spent a long time getting ready, wanting to look as good as possible. I wore some very colorful pants and a beautiful lime color silk blouse. I wore my wig, high heels and a nice bra so that I could leave open the top buttons of my blouse in order to reveal some cleavage.

When I arrived at the press conference, I stopped at the door for a few minutes and, being a little afraid, took some deep breaths. I walked towards the presentation room and saw him standing behind the podium. As soon as he realized that I had arrived, he immediately came over to greet me. We hugged each other with a lot of strength and love and talked for a little while until I went to sit because the press conference was about to start.

Although this launch was a work-related event, I went without anybody from my office that night because I thought I needed to start facing my new life without always depending on the company of others. Eventually, I realized that it was a very good decision because I began to recover my self-esteem from that moment on. Having to face my professional world—greeting and talking to people from the media whom I hadn't seen in several months—helped me to feel better and realize that life had gone on without me being a part of it and things had continued at the same pace as before I left. Each time somebody came up to me to compliment me on my new look, I felt that my ego was being massaged. All I could do was smile at the person and say, "Thank you." But immediately, I would think to myself, "If you only knew that this is a wig because I am totally bald."

At the end of the press conference, I went to the cock-tail party and started socializing. I realized that, even though I was going through something very difficult, life had kept going and I needed to leave my cave and try to integrate myself with reality. A couple of guys that I didn't know came up to talk to me. They gave me their business cards and asked if I would like to go out for a drink sometime. They had no idea what those invitations were doing to my ego or what I was going through at that time. I was feeling really happy and like a caught fish put back in water. After so many months of being sick, this was the first time I was really aware that life had gone on in my absence and I was feeling really happy to become part of it once again.

That night, with my ego totally massaged, I went home early, even though most of my friends continued to party at a restaurant. Although they had insisted that I joined them, I didn't want to overdo it my first time out. Somehow, I didn't want to burst the bubble that I was in. The following day, Javier and his producer, Gustavo, who also happened to be a very good friend of mine, called to invite me out for dinner. Since I didn't know they were going to be in Miami that particular weekend, I had already made plans with my friend, Carolina, since her daughter Angie was celebrating her birthday. We were going to take our children to the theater and to have dinner. I was starting to feel cheerful again and wanted my children to feel my good spirits, so I had to decline my friend's invitation, but asked them to join me for coffee after dinner. I truly enjoyed going out with Carolina and the children. Although the restaurant of her choice was very loud and service was slow, I felt pressed to get back home, where Javier and Gustavo would pick me up, as agreed. I wanted to change clothes, get rid of my bandana and wear my wig, in addition to touching up my makeup. When we left the restaurant, I got their call on my cell telling me that they were already waiting for me at my house. Bye-bye to the plan of changing clothes and fixing my makeup, I thought, but I told myself that it didn't really matter how I looked and should instead concentrate on the great time we were going to spend together as three old friends.

Since I hadn't planned that evening, I didn't make arrangements for a baby-sitter for my children. I called Sandra to ask her to take care of them. She came to pick them up and took them to her house for a sleepover. We greeted each other with a lot of affection and right away we started to talk and talk. We talked about a thousand different topics. A thousand memories came to our minds. We started to look at pictures of us from past years. Javier, Gustavo and I have known each other for such a long time and have shared so many special moments in different stages of our lives that we didn't get tired of talking, remembering those days and reliving those moments. The conversation was so interesting that we decided not to get out of my apartment. We prepared some hors d'oeuvres and drinks, and just sat in the living room.

During the first part of the evening, Javier was sitting on the sofa directly across from me. We were separated by the coffee table. The lighting in my apartment was soft. We could hear the water running from my little fountain. We had lit a lot of candles. The ambience was peaceful and true love and friendship could be felt among us. Several times I noticed Javier staring at me and pretended to ignore it. We were playing this flirting game that made me feel like a teenager falling in love with the most handsome guy from the football team.

Once we relaxed a little bit and after enjoying our talks for a couple of hours reliving memories with pictures, our conversation became much deeper. We talked about our personal relationships, affairs, disappointments with love and so on. Gustavo had noticed our flirting game. Looking directly at both Javier and me, he asked us if something had ever gone on between us. To tell the truth, his question was unexpected and caught me by surprise. For a moment, Javier and I just looked at each other, kind of thinking if anything had ever happened between us, and after a couple of seconds we both answered with a nostalgic and melancholic no.

After that question, Javier stood up, pulled one of my dining room chairs right next to me, and sat down. I felt a little nervous having him so close to me. I told them both that several times, particularly during my adolescence, I had dreamt that Javier was kissing me. I also told them that I had made this confession to Javier's girlfriend at the time, who happened to be my friend back then. For obvious reasons, she never liked my dreams. But I remember telling her just to make her jealous. Since those times I had felt attracted to him.

Gustavo couldn't believe what he just heard from me, especially since he knew from Javier himself that he had always felt the same way about me. Gustavo told me about the numerous times that Javier had told him that he had fantasized about me. All of a sudden, Gustavo stood up from his seat, picked up a microphone that I had next to my television, and pretended to be a reporter from a TV station, and began asking us questions about our feelings for each other. After each of our answers, he would then go back to the center of the living room and describe what that answer had represented in our lives. The game was very interesting and funny, especially because none of the three of us had realized that we were beginning to write a new chapter in our lives at that precise moment in time.

As we were listening to what Gustavo was saying, a beautiful feeling began to surround us. Javier was looking at me tenderly. In a very natural way, he held my hand, put it in between his hands, and began to kiss it very softly. I was very happy and excited, feeling like a 15-year-old that is being kissed for the very first time. Gustavo took his role of a television host very seriously. He kept asking us questions about our encounters throughout different stages in life. We would think about the answers for a second and respond, but our minds would just wander off.

The grasp of the hand led to caresses of the arm, which after a while led to an intense hug that, intermingled with deep stares, led to our first kiss, taking advantage of the moment when Gustavo left the room to go to the bathroom. That first kiss was long and beautiful, passionate but soft. At that moment, I felt transported to a new world. I remembered how many times I had imagined being with him like this. I totally forgot my physical condition, feeling extremely happy to be sharing the moment with him. He hugged me softly and whispered in my ear that he had loved me throughout the years and had also dreamed about that moment more than once. We were embroiled in this conversation when Gustavo came back to the living room and all he had to do was take a look at us to decide that it was time for him to leave. He asked for a telephone to call for a taxi.

Javier and I were totally happy and captivated by each other. We decided to get another drink and stepped out onto the balcony to enjoy the beautiful view. Out there, feeling the wind blow, we hugged and kissed again. I was overcome by a feeling of total happiness because at that moment I had begun to feel and live again.

From my terrace we could see that the taxi Gustavo called for had arrived. Gustavo went inside my apartment to pick up his briefcase and Javier held me once again. Looking directly into my eyes, Javier asked me if I wanted him to leave or to stay with me. I thought about the answer for a split second and, looking at him in the same way, I asked him to stay with me. We said goodbye to Gustavo. The two of us were alone now.

Without getting too intimate into my personal life, I can honestly write that that evening had been one of the most wonderful of my life. Neither my bald head, nor my overweight, nor the scars all over my body, nor my illness were an obstacle for him to love me. The pure and profound love that we have felt for each other throughout the years was demonstrated that night when he made me his. We made love all night long. I felt very much a part of him, as if we had been together forever. He didn't stop telling me how beautiful I was. He would even kiss my bald head, telling me that hair wasn't important to him because he loved the soul of the woman I was. That night I felt what true love is between two souls that found one another in this life and continued to love each other despite time and distance.

After a couple of hours of sleep, I woke up the next morning wanting to make sure that he was really there and that it wasn't just a beautiful dream. I couldn't believe what had happened. When I saw him laying down next to me, I had to pinch myself several times just to make sure that what had happened was real. I felt so good. I knew that his love was real and pure. Our time together was the best medicine life could have offered me at that precise moment. That incredible experience has been, without a doubt, one of the most beautiful moments of my existence.

I was lying down next to him, relaxing and feeling fully content, when he woke up. He looked at me, smiled, and said that waking up next to me made him very happy.

We talked for a little while before he left, realizing we were still captivated by the magic that entrapped us the night before. Feelings and emotions were so strong and intense that we didn't want to let go of each other. We didn't want to be apart. Both of us would have wanted that night not to end so soon and for the morning not to have begun.

Needless to say, we lived a fairytale weekend. It was an extraordinary experience for both of us. But for me, due to my circumstances, it was the best that could have happened. I discovered that true love not only withstands the test of time, but also that physical appearance is not an obstacle for its expression. Besides being a unique experience, it helped me because it made me feel like a woman. No medication could have healed my self-esteem the way that weekend did. When, after three days, the time came for him to leave, he left in Miami a new woman who felt alive again.

Saying goodbye was easy since we both entered into this experience knowing that, even though we love each other very much, our relationship wasn't going to be permanent because we live very different lives. Even knowing that, I didn't care about taking risks for the first time in a long while. I decided to live a moment that was probably never going to repeat itself, because life goes on and changes as do people and circumstances.

Once he left, I felt at peace with myself and was very happy. His presence in my life during that Difficult Journey gave me a lot of confidence that I had been lacking for some time and needed very much. From that moment on, I felt beautiful, attractive and loved once again. Above all, I realized that, even though cancer had altered my body, it hadn't changed my soul. As of that weekend, I felt like a true woman again.

ON MY WAY TO RADIATION

Seven months had passed since I was first diagnosed with breast cancer. To be honest, I was very anxious to begin my radiation therapy because I knew that it would represent the closing of my healing cycle.

When my clinical oncologist advised me that it was time to look for a radiologist, I did so. Both she and my friend Tito, the pathologist, recommended the same doctor. I called his office and made an appointment to see him. On that first call, the receptionist transferred me to the office manager who, in a very abrupt way, informed me that I needed to come to my first consultation with $300 which I had to pay before the doctor saw me. I thought her attitude was very rude but that maybe she was having a bad day and took it out on me. The truth is I didn't give it much importance because I was looking forward to having my first appointment with a radiologist two weeks later.

At that time in my life, I was feeling better emotionally, but financially I was in a very bad situation. Up to that point I owed more than $150,000 in medical expenses. For the first time since I began with this problem, I started to worry about my financial situation. My father was helping me out with some of the bills. Two of my aunts had loaned me some money and one of my uncles was paying for my children's school tuition. But even with all that help, my medical debt was extremely high, considering that I wasn't able to work quite yet and had to keep sustaining my children and my house. Suddenly, I opened my eyes and realized that I was in a very difficult financial situation.

The day of my appointment arrived and I went full of hope because I honestly felt that I was approaching the final leg in my fight for life. When I got to the doctor's office, which was located in a building next to the hospital, I again felt that strange sensation of being in a place where I never thought I would be. The big signs announcing the entrance to the oncology and radiation unit gave me the chills. That feeling of doubt and uncertainty came over me again. I stopped for a second, stared at the signs, and told myself that it was OK, that I was at the end of the treatment, and that I needed to be strong to be able to continue with it. Even with this positive thinking, I felt pretty sad and couldn't help my eyes from filling with tears once again. I took a deep breath and walked into his office.

The receptionist welcomed me to the office, gave me a questionnaire to fill out, and indicated to me that I needed to see the office manager before seeing the doctor. When I walked into her office and greeted her, I quickly realized that this woman, named Sandy, was quite a bitter person. She stared at me from head to toe. Without even getting up from her chair, she asked me for the $300. I looked at her with a bit of surprise because I thought she was kind of rude. She proceeded to tell me that it was their policy to charge their patients in advance just in case they decided not to do the treatments right there. She emphasized that if I decided not to stay with that doctor and look for another place for my treatments, they were not going to be without their payment. She reiterated that my payment was required before going in to meet the doctor. A little upset and without really believing what I was hearing, I told her that I had never paid a doctor before meeting with him and that I wasn't about to do it then. I assured her that I would stop by to pay before leaving the office, but after my appointment with him. We discussed about it for a few minutes, each defending her own position, until at last, with a very mean attitude, she let me go in to see the doctor, but not before warning me not to try to escape through the back door without paying. After that comment I felt very bad. I was about to run from that place and go home but didn't do it because I knew I had to see the doctor. I just took a deep breath and walked into the waiting room. "What a rude attitude this woman has," I thought to myself. But I also realized that I shouldn't judge the whole medical team simply because of the office manager's attitude. I sat down and waited to be called.

A few minutes later a nurse came to take me to yet another waiting room. Even though I was trying not to think about the experience with Sandy, it wouldn't leave my mind. Her comments made me feel disgusted, particularly at that time when I was very vulnerable. Sitting down waiting to be seen by the doctor, I realized that the only time I had previously spoken to Sandy was over the phone and her attitude had been just as mean. She was a difficult person with very little sympathy. For the first time since I started my fight against cancer, I faced a person who was part of a medical team who was inconsiderate and lacked compassion.

Having waited for more than an hour, a nurse came to ask me to take off my clothes because she was going to examine me. As it is customary in hospitals, the room was very cold, so I wore the gown she gave me. After asking me all the questions from a questionnaire and taking my vital signs, she took a couple of pictures of the area where I had the surgeries. She left the room, leaving me there by myself again for a long time. So many things were coming to my mind; so many questions I kept asking myself. I still couldn't believe that I was sitting there going through all of this. It was a very difficult situation.

The doctor came to see me at last. Things didn't work out very well with him either. He greeted me in a hurry and started asking me questions. He wouldn't even let me finish giving him the answers when he would interrupt me with the next question. I felt a little bit uncomfortable and found it rather unusual that he took two telephone calls while reviewing my files and asking me questions. By listening to his conversations, I found out that he was going on vacation the following week. It bothered me that he was trying to arrange who would be taking care of his house while he and his family were away because I thought he wasn't respecting my time as a patient. Once again I thought that maybe I was overly sensitive. I tried to make some sense of the situation by thinking that a phone call under normal circumstances would have been OK. But at that moment it was annoying me.

After he talked to me for a little bit and examined my scars, I told him that I was very interested in having him as my radiologist because two of his colleagues had recommended him very strongly. I also explained to him that I hadn't been working for awhile and didn't have medical insurance. I asked him if I could work out a payment plan with his office in a way that would be comfortable to me because the most important thing at that time was to be able to receive treatment. I don't know if he didn't understand what I had just told him, because maybe he was too consumed with planning his vacation. Without giving me any answers, he stood up, gave me an appointment to see him again 10 days later and, before walking out of the room, asked me to go see Sandy before leaving the office because

I needed to take care of my bill for that day. His comment hit me like a rock. That doctor was simply concerned about his money. How sad.

Once he left the room and I started putting my clothes back on, I had these mixed feelings of frustration, anger and disillusionment. How many problems would I have avoided if I only had health insurance? During my journey I had learned to be humble and accept my difficult financial situation. But it still was beyond my understanding how some people could be so insensitive. I felt that I was in a place where I was just another number to them. They didn't understand that I was a woman fighting to recover my health and my life.

Obviously, I went to see Sandy before leaving the doctor's office and paid her for the appointment. I got into my car, started driving toward my house, and just started crying while on the expressway. I couldn't believe the lack of compassion I had faced at that office. I couldn't believe that this group of people was so selfish. For the first time since I had been diagnosed, I had run into some medical personnel who were selfish and lacked humanity. It was very hard for me to understand it because up until then I had learned that cancer is an illness that teaches us the meaning of the word compassion. I was in a very serious predicament because I certainly didn't feel at ease with this doctor, but I knew that he was my only choice if I wanted to get financial help from the hospital. I was very confused. I needed to put my thoughts in order, put my feelings aside, and become more objective.

The next day I received a fax with the estimate of what the radiation treatment would cost me. On the fax it stated that if I wanted to receive treatment from them, I needed to pay half of the total amount on the day of my next appointment. The bill was $9,800 for the services of the doctor and his staff. That didn't include X-rays, technicians, tests or the radiation itself. The fee was only for the doctor and his assistants. I was totally shocked. I knew I needed to receive the treatment because it was the final leg of my healing process. But it was a lot of money that they needed in advance and I simply didn't have it at that time. The feeling of helplessness that I felt for several days after that was overwhelming. I needed time to think about how I was going to get the money to cover such a high expense.

A few days later after reviewing my financial situation, looking for money here and there, and asking for help, I called Sandy to try to make another kind of payment arrangement with them. In a way that felt somewhat sarcastic, she told me that my only other choice was to make two payments for the total amount, one at the beginning of the treatment and the other at the end. She emphasized that if I didn't have the cash or credit cards to be able to cover the payments, she suggested that I should start looking for another doctor that would better fit my budget. She then told me that if it was hard for me to find a doctor I could afford, I should consider going to the county hospital and simply wait a few months to receive treatment. After that comment I couldn't take it anymore. Trying to pretend that I wasn't crying, I told her again that this was a very large amount of money. I asked her if they only care for wealthy patients. What about those who don't have the money available and need to get treatment? What would they do? She simply answered by saying that people without money or medical insurance seek the help of other doctors or go to the county hospital. She told me one more time that there was nothing else I could do. She suggested that, if I wasn't able to get the money, I needed to let her know within 24 hours because she couldn't hold my appointment since the waiting list of people seeking treatment with them was extremely long.

Frustration, pain, sadness, anger ... everything that I was experiencing at that time was so overwhelming that I felt like an extremely insignificant human being, totally consumed by the situation. On the one hand, I knew that I needed to stay with this doctor if I wanted to get some financial help from the hospital. On the other, I was totally disappointed at the way these people were treating me. It was a very uncomfortable situation. I honestly did not want to be treated by this doctor, but having made the arrangements with the hospital to get some help through their charity wasn't that easy. I had spent a lot of time pursuing it and was aware that it wasn't going to be easy for me to get this kind of help from any other place. It was very hard for me to accept the fact that money could play such an important role at this stage of my healing process. I was not asking the doctor to perform some kind of plastic surgery. I was begging him for the opportunity to receive the radiation treatment that would prevent the cancer from returning. I was feeling very bad and helpless to be in this situation. I was very angry with Sandy and found it hard to understand how a relatively young woman could be so mean with somebody who was so sick, when I was only trying to fight for my life. I felt sorry for her and wondered how much bitterness and frustration was inside that fat body of hers.

I was in the middle of these thoughts when my friend Carolina came to visit me. She noticed that I was very worried. I told her what had just happened. Her eyes filled with tears. She hugged me and offered to call her dad in Germany to ask him for a personal loan so that I could borrow the money and finish my treatment. Her noble gesture reminded me one more time that the world is full of good people who are trying to help us. The fact that I had found a group of money-grubbers didn't mean that my treatment was going to stop. As the saying goes, "When one door closes, another opens." I knew that somehow I was going to be able to find the money I needed.

Luckily, it wasn't necessary to call Carolina's dad since I was able to get my father to help me. Although he had helped me with some of my bills, this was a large amount of money even for him. But he asked me to fax him the estimate because somehow he was going to help me come up with the money so that I could start my treatment. Fortunately, he did it. Fifteen days later and after a serious setback, I was able to start receiving my radiation treatment. I am very grateful to my father for his help.

UNEXPECTED SETBACK

"Last night my mommy came home from having dinner with a friend. When she came home she felt really, really bad. She kept pressing her stomach and made painful expressions with her face. I gave my mommy a massage because she usually likes them, but after I had just started she asked me to stop. I was scared because she always enjoys my massages. Her friend Rey called my mom and five minutes later came over to the house with his friend Phil who is a doctor. They came to see her. Rey came into my room and told my sister and me that Phil was a doctor, but Izzy jumped on the bed face down and started to cry and cry. The two of us were very afraid, but Phil told us that it seemed that my mom had kidney stones, so he had to take her to the hospital. We told her that we have a neighbor that has a wheelchair, so we went to ask if we could borrow it so we could take my mommy to the car. Phil and Rey went with my mommy to the hospital and we stayed home with Adela. After a little while, Phil called to let us know that my mommy had to stay in the hospital because they needed to run some tests. I am very worried for my mommy."

— *Tommy*

It was Tuesday night and I was very happy because, after several months, I was going out again to have dinner with my friend Andrew. I met him when I first moved to Miami and began a beautiful friendship. We both like sushi and usually went out for it at least twice a month. I missed those dinners very much during the time I was sick because they had become a sort of tradition for us. We loved exploring new restaurants. Even though I still wasn't allowed to eat any sushi due to my low cell count, Andrew invited me to a fancy restaurant located relatively close to my house to celebrate that I had finished chemotherapy and was getting very close to beginning the last leg of my treatments.

I had a stomach ache that whole day but didn't give it too much importance because I assumed it was just a side effect from chemotherapy. But while we were having dinner at the restaurant, the pain became very strong to a point where I had to tell Andrew that we needed to skip desert because I needed him to take me back home. He was worried about my health. Trying to make it seem less important, he suggested I go to the bathroom to relieve my gases in order to feel better.

He drove me to my apartment building. I walked all the way to the elevator, got inside, and went up to my floor. When the elevator door opened, I couldn't even take one step. The pain was very intense. I managed to walk into my home, said hello to my kids, and went straight to my bedroom and laid down on my bed. I began doing my breathing exercises trying to relax and mentally distance myself from the pain, but it wasn't working.

The pain was so intense that I asked Adela to talk to Rey to ask him to call our friend Phil, a pediatrician acquaintance of ours who lived in the building, to see if he could come up to examine me. Fifteen minutes later they were both in my apartment. Phil began to examine me and asked my children to leave my room. He decided it was necessary to contact my urologist/oncologist because his first thought was that it was something related to my kidney. Both doctors talked to each other over the phone and decided that the best solution was to take me to the hospital because they suspected many things but weren't sure what was causing such pain. When Phil told me that he needed to take me to the hospital, I agreed because the pain was very intense.

Once again I started to think about the new expense that this would represent.

There was a lot of commotion at home. Of course, my children were very worried. While we were waiting for the doctors' decision, Tommy sat behind me and began rubbing my back, telling me constantly how much he loved me. I was very grateful to him because I usually enjoy his massages, but the pain was so intense that even that nice massage felt uncomfortable. Tommy looked at me. With fear in his eyes, he asked me if I was going to die. Phil overheard him, sat down next to him, and explained to him that it seemed that I had a kidney stone as a result of the chemotherapy. He told him that when that happens it is painful rather than dangerous. Tommy felt a little better after hearing that explanation.

My children were able to get me a wheelchair from our next-door neighbor. With the help of Rey and Phil, I sat down on it and they wheeled me to the car to take me to the hospital. My children stayed at home with Adela. They were both very worried, but I knew that they were going to feel protected with Adela in charge.

The pain was extremely intense. I felt it right in the middle of my stomach. During the whole ride to the hospital, Phil was holding my hand while praying to God, asking him to give me strength to withstand the pain. I really liked his faith and felt very protected and safe with him.

Once I got to the hospital, they took me to the emergency room where doctors began to examine me. After a little while, my friends started arriving. Adela had decided to tell everybody about my setback. After staying with me past midnight, Phil left, but not before he talked to the doctors in charge, asking them to take special care of me. Sandra stayed with me for a while. She told me that Antonio was outside waiting to see me. We were still waiting for the results of the test they had performed on me, but it seemed that it was a kidney stone.

Even though the pain was still very intense, they couldn't give me any painkillers until they determined what my problem was. Sandra had called my parents to let them know that I had to be admitted to the hospital. She didn't have any more details to give them. They were feeling quite worried and I asked her to keep them informed.

It was almost dawn. I asked Sandra to go home because I was worried that with her pregnancy she would get very tired. Once she left my room, Antonio came in to see me. He did not leave my side for the next 48 hours.

The pain was extremely intense and I had started to vomit. Approximately every 10 minutes, I felt a strong spasm that would force me to clench my stomach and make me throw up. Antonio would put the spit tray in front of my mouth and hold my back while I threw up. As soon as I was finished, he would kindly clean my face. We spent several hours like this until at last a doctor came to give me the results of the tests. It was not a kidney stone but an intestinal occlusion. At that time they didn't know if they could perform a special treatment to open it up or if I needed to undergo yet another surgery. I was very afraid at the news and asked Antonio to call my parents and let them know what was going on.

After so many hours, they were finally able to give me some painkillers. The pain eased off after a couple of hours. I thought that maybe the problem had gone away and my intestine had opened up by itself. I was hoping that they were going to let me go home soon. While I was thinking about that, a new doctor came in, introduced himself, and told me they were taking me to a private room to keep me under close supervision during the start of my treatment. My room was inside the hospital's oncology unit.

Besides reducing my pain, the sedatives I was getting kept me half-asleep, helping me to rest a little bit. I had been up for more than 24 hours straight. Every time I opened my eyes, I realized that Antonio was there by my side keeping me company. The poor guy was very tired but he wouldn't leave my side. Only if somebody else came to stay with me did he leave my room to drink coffee or have something to eat. That same day they put a tube through my nose with a very long plastic piece that extended to the back of my nasal passage right down into my stomach. The tube they had to tape to my face was very thick and uncomfortable. I looked pretty bad. In addition to being totally bald with huge dark circles under my eyes, I looked very pale. For the first time during my illness it wasn't pleasant for me to receive visits under those circumstances. The long tube that went through my nose and reached my stomach was constantly pumping out a green yellowish substance into a clear jar placed next to my bed that didn't look good at all. That hospital stay was very uncomfortable, not only for me but also for those who visited me, because nobody likes to see a loved one looking so sick and undergoing so much pain.

On the second day I was in the hospital, my father told Antonio he was flying out to see how he could help me. Antonio told me that my dad sounded really worried about me and kept calling to ask about my condition every so often. Despite all the hardships I endured during this Difficult Journey, I am certain that the coming together of my father and me during this process was very important for my healing, physically as well as spiritually.

The second day went by very slowly. I was extremely uncomfortable with all those tubes, even though the sedatives kept me more or less asleep. That night an orderly came to take me to a very cold and kind of dark room in the hospital's basement where the treatment to try to open the intestine was going to be administered. The treatment was horrible and painful. They had to put radioactive substance inside the tube that I had in my nose and push it down really hard so it would dye my intestines. Then, they would lie me down under a huge X-ray machine. While all of this was taking place, the technicians kept talking about their personal lives. I was feeling lost and very uncomfortable. On top of my feeling really sick, the room was extremely cold and they had only given me a small sheet to use to cover myself. They were not allowed to let me leave the room until they found the exact cause of my problem. I spent more than 5 hours in that room. The painkillers stopped working after the first two hours and I began to feel the same intense pain that I had felt before. Not only was I feeling physically sick, I was also afraid and felt very lonely. The X-ray technicians would come to me, make a small comment, and leave the room again. I would have long periods of time spent totally alone. Anguish began to overcome me. That was one of the most difficult nights of my sickness. To be very honest, moments existed during which the pain, exhaustion and cold made me think that I was dying. That night I felt very strongly that my body just wanted to take a break. I began to give up. I couldn't keep fighting anymore.

After pleading several times with the radiologist and after seeing me suffering with the intense pain for so long, he agreed to get me some more sedatives. Once they gave them to me, I fell into a deep sleep. All I can remember is opening my eyes while being wheeled into my room and looking at Lilia, who had replaced Antonio as my bed-sitter. She was going to spend the night with me at the hospital. She hugged me, held my hand, and realized that I was feeling terribly sick. She began to transfer energy to me with her hands and helped me to meditate and to try to relax. I felt happy to have her by my side. Even though we had met right after my surgeries, I felt that she was being like a protective mother to me during the whole period of sickness.

The following day my dad arrived at the hospital. I noticed that he was totally shocked to see me in such a bad physical appearance. Besides the tubes in my nose, I had several IVs in both arms, which were full of bruises. Despite all this, I was very glad to see my dad next to me because I felt protected one more time. I know that for him, the fact of staying with me during those days at the hospital was very difficult. He felt uncomfortable and sad looking at me under those circumstances. Even though he tried to spend as much time as he could with me, he would use any excuse to leave my room to go drink some coffee, get the newspaper, or simply stretch his legs. Like a true man, he wasn't very comfortable at the hospital.

Tommy and Izzy were very worried about me. They called me on the phone several times during the day. They noticed that my voice wasn't as strong and happy as usual. I sounded weak and in pain. Nevertheless, they were happy to talk to me and to learn that I was trying to recuperate from this setback so I could be home with them again. Against my wishes, Tommy's father took him to the hospital to see me. Even though I had asked him not to bring Tommy to see me because I didn't like my children to see me looking so bad, he ignored my request. Suddenly, there was my little son, next to my bed, avoiding my eyes because he was very impressed to see me all tubed up. It is very difficult for children to understand and accept the physical pain of a parent.

My stay at the hospital wasn't easy. The pain was going away slowly but surely. After six days and two very painful treatments, they let me go home at last. It wasn't necessary to do surgery on me, but when I left the hospital they put me on a very strict diet. I was somehow excited about leaving the hospital because I knew that finally I was going to start my radiation therapy, which had to be postponed due to this unforeseen setback.

RADIATION

"My mommy just started radiation a little while ago. Radiation is as if they shoot rays at your skin and it burns. My mommy's skin has been red as a tomato for the last week and it burns her a little bit, but she doesn't complain because she is very strong. She told me that radiation is the last part of her cancer problem and she says it is the easiest one because it doesn't hurt when they burn her."

— *Tommy*

"My mom's booby and the part under her arm are purple, but you cannot see them unless she shows them to you. At least her hair is starting to grow now and when she comes out of the shower, her hair is all spiky and she looks really funny."

— *Izzy*

Once I left the hospital after my unforeseen setback, I contacted the radiologist's office to reschedule my appointment for radiation therapy. I still didn't have the almost $5,000 that I needed to pay before I could start my therapy, but I figured I would use my credit cards while I was waiting for the money from my father. Upon arriving at the doctor's office on the day of my appointment, Sandy took me into her private office. I can honestly say that it seemed she was enjoying the fact that my first payment had to be divided among three different credit cards. Looking back at it, I can only say that it was very unpleasant having to work with her, but I understand now that we can learn even from bad, selfish or jealous people.

They did what is called a "simulator" on that first day. During the simulator, the doctor and technician measure the area in which the patient is going to receive the radiation. They also determine the exact position in which the patient has to be while getting the treatment. They take some X-rays to verify that the marks they paint on the skin coincide with the areas to be radiated.

I had been told that it was very important for the doctor to be present on that day because he was going to be the one who eventually would determine and verify the measurements for my radiation. I laid down on the stretcher waiting for the doctor for almost one hour, but he didn't show up. The room in which I was waiting was very cold. I asked the technician to give me a blanket because it was a long wait. When he came back to give me the blanket, he told me that the doctor was busy and was not coming to see me. But he assured me that he would give him my file and recommendations personally to get his approval for the treatment. I felt a little let down thinking that the relationship with patients at this doctor's office was much less than I was expecting. Once again, I realized that the radiologist didn't care about my health. He only cared about my wallet. How sad. I believed that my displeasure showed because the technician felt very sorry and tried to give me a thousand excuses for why the doctor wouldn't come to see me.

Not having to wait for the doctor any longer, the simulator began. The technician would measure very meticulously the area on my breast where I had the tumor. Then he would paint it with some color markers and place on my breast a special kind of adhesive tape with some type of wires. I had to lay down very still while he would walk out of the room to take some X-rays. The simulator lasted for about two hours, during which he would do the same procedure over and over again. When we finished, I left the office with a new appointment to do another simulator the following week. It was a little bit strange to look at my breast after that visit to the radiologist. It was all painted with thick green and blue lines in addition to having the tape with the wires stuck to my skin. The technician had told me that I had to be very careful while taking a shower because I needed to come back a week later with the paint and the wires still in place. I felt weird having all that stuff on my breast. It looked very unattractive but I wasn't worried about it since I wasn't about to show off my breast to anybody at the time.

As soon as I left the radiologist's office, I went straight to a very nice lingerie store at the shopping mall. The nurse had suggested that during the radiation period I should only wear cotton bras. I decided to spoil myself and bought three that I would use during the 45 days of this treatment.

The following week I went back for the second part of the simulator. On that day, besides measuring me and taking X-rays of my breast, they also did some small tattoos in the main places where I was going to be getting the treatment. The technician explained to me that the tattoos were permanent but are so tiny that they seemed like little birthmarks strategically placed on my breasts and my side. I had to go back one more time after this visit just to make sure that everything was all right before the treatment began.

The first days of radiation were easy. Leaving my house early in the morning to drive the 25 miles to the hospital took more effort than the treatment itself. In reality, the only way to know that one has been receiving radiation treatment is because the skin changes color and is more sensitive as the days go by. While getting the radiation, you don't feel or see anything. You simply have to lie down in the stretcher without moving at all for several minutes while listening to the machine turning on and off until you can hear the technician's voice through the speakers informing you that the session has ended.

The kind of cancer that I was fighting required 33 doses on my breast and seven doses on my side where they had removed the lymph nodes. The doses were administered at the same time each day, Monday to Friday. It is easy to say forty doses, but after the first 10, I began to feel some side effects.

During the two months of radiation treatment, my days would go by pretty much the same way. I would leave my house and drive straight to the hospital every morning. Once there, I would give my car to the parking attendant outside the office. After registering, I would proceed to the dressing room where I undressed from the waist up and put on a hospital gown. Then, I sat down in a waiting area along with several women under similar circumstances and waited for my turn. Sandra would accompany me on the great majority of the days. We would use the driving time to chat about different topics and countdown the days left for the both of us to be finished with our respective situations.

Since the appointments were Monday to Friday at the same time and each patient had more or less the same schedule, I would find myself in the waiting area with the same ladies. At the beginning, we would look at each other and simply say hello. As time passed, we began having more profound conversations about our lives, symptoms and experiences. After all, we were all partners in the same pain and somehow fighting the same battle. From this group of patients I learned a lot. I especially realized the importance of having a positive attitude towards such a big adversity.

During these sessions I got to meet people with much smaller problems than mine as well as others in very grave situations. I realized that cancer is an illness that attacks indiscriminately. It makes no distinctions between sex, age, social status or anything. It is a terrible and treacherous illness that gushes forth from the deepest part of the body of those of us who are susceptible to it. In a secretive way and without warning, it starts growing and spreading until one day we find out that we have it, changing our lives forever. From the information I gathered from all those women during that period of time, I found out that none of them suspected its existence and it caught practically all of us by surprise.

It was a fascinating experience to talk to each and every one of these women awaiting treatment in the same room with me. Among other things, I realized that the insecurity and incredulity that this illness brings out were common feelings. I understood that the process of accepting the problem follows certain steps that are similar for everyone: first there is doubt, fear and confusion; then, anguish and anger; and, finally, the process of acceptance and the fight to survive. We were all in exactly this part of the process, even though some of the cases were worse than mine. We were all getting radiation treatment in the hope that the cancer would not manifest itself again.

After a few days, we all said goodbye to the first lady among us who was finishing her treatment. That was just the first of many celebrations we had during the seven weeks of my treatment. Each time one of us "graduated," the others would celebrate the occasion.

Three weeks prior to finishing my radiation therapy, Sandra gave birth to a beautiful baby girl, Aleksa. Since she had been by my side during all these months, I was very privileged to have been with her in the delivery room and be able to welcome such a beautiful baby into the world. It was a very moving experience that led me to question the greatness of life for several days. On one side I was fighting with all of my strength to be able to destroy that terrible disease because I wanted to live, but on the other I had in front of me this beautiful brand new baby, defenseless and very small, with a long life ahead of her. As you can imagine, the birth of Aleksa was reason to celebrate along with my entire group of radiology patients, because Sandra had also become a friend with most of them. They were all very anxious to see the new baby come onto this world. I guess that, to a lot of them, the birth of a new life represented new hope for all of us.

Our routine was pretty much the same everyday. I would get to the doctor's office every morning. In the dressing room, I had the opportunity to chat with all of the ladies. Then, a nurse would come to take me to the room where I would receive my treatment. Mondays and Thursdays were terrifying for me because on those days they had to weigh me before getting the treatment. During the radiation period I gained a few pounds, which I really didn't like at all. Inside the treatment room, I would lay down on the stretcher under the X-ray machine. The technician would proceed to remove my robe and position the X-ray machine, pointing it right to the spot where I had been previously marked. I had to lie still for 10 or 15 minutes in a rather uncomfortable position, with my left hand tied up above my head and without being able to make the slightest movement. Once I achieved the ideal position, the nurse and the technician would leave the room to begin administering the radiation. I was there all by myself with that very intimidating piece of equipment. Everyday I would take advantage of the situation to pray to the Holy Mother and the Supreme Being, as well as to my guardian angels, asking them to bathe me in their light.

I invoked them to offer me through those healing rays the cure my body needed to rid itself of the error that had been produced in it and to heal completely. It's funny, but I was able to find a very special peace around me. Even though the room was very cold and intimidating, I felt at ease and peace with myself. Somehow, I felt protected spiritually. That's exactly how I felt at that time. I am lucky that I was able to receive my radiation therapy with a positive attitude every day.

My relationship with those who had to administer the treatment to me every day was very good. The technicians, nurses and supervisors were good people who knew how to make this journey a little less difficult. They all made me feel important every day by saying good morning with a big smile and calling me by first name, an opposite attitude completely contrary to that of the people who worked for my radiation doctor. Once again, I found in the hospital staff the pleasant treatment, love, compassion, and a wide variety of noble feelings that have characterized the special people whom I have found during my sickness. I am very grateful to them and to a lot of others for helping me to walk this last leg of my fight against cancer.

I was very fortunate to have been surrounded by friends all throughout my surgeries, doctors' appointments and chemotherapies. I decided to take advantage of Aleksa's birth to try to go alone to the radiation therapy. Somehow, I wanted to feel that, slowly but surely, I was regaining my independence. I would take advantage of my daily drive to the hospital to listen to some motivational tapes that a friend of mine had given me. I also wanted to use this time to put my ideas in order, to dream and plan the future, to listen to music, and simply to feel free.

My trips to the hospital alone ended up being very few because I wasn't feeling very well physically toward the last part of my treatment. I was very nauseated and extremely tired. On top of it all, my skin was chapped and burned. I was uncomfortable and in pain. Once again, I was very grateful for the kindness of my friends who would take the time to go with me to the hospital. I am very fortunate in that respect. My friends, whom I now consider to be my spiritual family, didn't want me to go through this alone. There was never a lack of volunteers to accompany me on my trips to the hospital.

By the second week of radiation, my blood count began to deteriorate rapidly. The doctor ordered a blood check every other day. After being through all those surgeries and chemotherapy, a blood test should have been very simple, but it wasn't like that. At that time, I was very tired and uncomfortable with the whole situation. Something as simple as a blood test would bother me. It was also very tiring mentally to hear the nurse every single day telling me that my blood count was getting worse every day and that treatment would have to be suspended if it continued going downhill. I had to call the hospital almost every day before leaving the house the find out whether or not the treatment could be administered. Even though my platelets were down to 30,000 units (the average is 140,000 to 170,000), the doctor never suspended the treatment. What I did notice is that I started bruising all over my body very easily and didn't really feel like doing anything all day. The nausea, the change in my pallet and the tiredness were constant day in and day out. I mentioned it to the doctor during one of the very few times that he tended to me, but I got the impression that he didn't give my situation much importance. The very first time I met with him he told me that he would be present during the simulator and give me a checkup once a week to make sure everything went along as it should. We now know that he wasn't there for the simulator and that he sent a substitute doctor on three out of the seven weeks that he was supposed to see me. I was particularly upset on my last appointment with him. Since it was my last day, I was full of questions. I wanted to know his opinion about my health and what to expect from now on in my life. The doctor happened to be on vacation again and the nurse was the one who gave me the instructions about what to do with my skin during the following days at home. She was the one that gave me a certificate of completion once I finished the treatment. I really didn't like that the doctor wasn't there with me. I disliked it even more when the nurse told me on my last visit that she was going to give me an appointment for the doctor to give me a check up two weeks later, making it clear that this appointment was not included in the price they had already given me and that it was an additional expense which had to be paid on that visit.

On one of the very few times that I was able to meet with the doctor, I talked to him about Sandy, his office manager, and expressed my concern for the lack of sensitivity of all his staff. He looked at me for a moment and told me that he was sorry about my perception. He suggested that I send him my comments in writing so he could keep them in a file. He also told me that I shouldn't take it personally because I needed to understand that to them this was just a business and they treated it as such. I was totally shocked.

During the radiation period, I tried to resume some of my everyday activities. I was thrilled when I was able to drive my car to pick up my children from school again. I would take advantage after returning home in the afternoon to rest and take a nap. Although I wanted to do a lot of things, what I thought I could do was more than what I could really do physically. On one occasion, I asked Tom to take care of the children for the whole weekend. I did not even get out of bed during those two whole days. All

I did that weekend was rest, sleep, rest and sleep. I was extremely tired.

Once the fourth week of treatment had begun, my skin began to burn and it hurt a lot. At first, the area that was being radiated turned very red as if I had been under the sun without any protection during the whole day. As the days passed, the red turned into purple. I got a lot of blisters and my skin got slightly infected. When that happened, I stopped wearing a bra and would simply wear big cotton T-shirts that wouldn't touch my skin. But having skin like that did not prevent me from continuing the treatment. They simply gave me some antibiotics to prevent a bigger infection. Having my skin burned was very painful. Being like that made me think about how much suffering people who get burned on several parts of their bodies must endure. That helped me realize how fortunate I was because I knew that my burns were going to last for a short period of time since my skin was going to heal rapidly once the treatment was finished. It is incredible how wise nature is.

Seven weeks are easy to say. But when one is undergoing a medical treatment such as that one, seven weeks are only part of A Difficult Journey. Out of all my experiences during my illness, the time of radiation was the strangest. On one hand, I was glad to have arrived at this stage of my healing process. On the other, the lack of human interest from my radiology doctor and his staff opened my eyes to a harsh and insensitive reality. Even though during the whole process I had come upon extraordinary, good and passionate doctors, I encountered a doctor that had forgotten the fundamental basics of medicine. He reminded me that, unfortunately, we live in a society in which money can make people forget about the fundamental rights of life.

GIFTS FROM THE SOUL

One of the things that surprised me the most during this healing process is the spirituality of people around me. It has been incredible to realize what an important role faith plays in the recovery process. It is really important to understand that, no matter how difficult a situation can be, everything happens for a reason. It doesn't matter what our faith is as long as we believe that there is a Supreme Being.

During my Difficult Journey, the encouragement, strength and support that people gave me were very rewarding. To help me continue my fight, people would share with me their own personal experiences or those they knew of others close to them that they believed to be miraculous or extraordinarily positive. In addition to their anecdotes, a lot of people shared with me their faith and beliefs, with the purpose of inspiring me in my long journey. Although the majority of the experiences they shared with me had happy endings, it wasn't always the case.

For several days Sandra was very excited about the visit of one her best friends from Peru who was the daughter of a breast cancer patient. Sandra really wanted me to meet her friend, thinking it might help me to talk to her to learn the feelings and emotions that a daughter of a mother with breast cancer experienced while growing up. When they were both teenagers, her friend's mother had been diagnosed with cancer. She thought that I could share her experiences and compare them with my daughter's. I was really looking forward to meet with her friend. We had lunch and a nice conversation. After telling me how she dealt with this issue for 10 years while her mother was fighting her disease, I asked her how her mother was doing then. When I asked that question they looked at each other and didn't know exactly how to answer. Sandra had forgotten to tell me that her friend's mother had lost her battle to cancer a couple of months before. When they explained her passing away right in the middle of the conversation, it was very hard for me to take.

The first time I told my friend Rey that I had cancer, he pulled out his wallet and took out a little stamp of Jesus. He showed it to me, telling me that it was old and not in the best condition because he had been carrying it with him since he was a teenager. He said it was very special to him. Every time he was worried about or afraid of something, he would take it out from his wallet, hold it in his hands, and pray. He then looked at me, put the stamp in my hands, and told me that from that moment on the image was going to be protecting me as much as it had protected him throughout the years. He felt that it would do me some good to keep it.

When I went with my dad to Texas, he gave me a holy cross that had been blessed by Pope John Paul II. It is a beautiful silver cross. What made it even more beautiful was his gesture of giving it to me. As far as I knew, my father had never been very religious. It felt good to know that, in moments of anguish and pain, even he can have faith in God.

One certain Sunday around noon, I had the visit from a friend with whom I've had some differences. She had heard about my problem and talked to her mother about it. Her mother, who lives in New York, is a very religious woman and a follower of this particular church that has some holy water known to have healed a lot of sick people. She had gone to this church to get a bottle of holy water for me.

During my recovery, my friend Aida had gone on vacation to Portugal. When she came back, she gave me a little bottle of holy water from Fatima, along with a small statue of the virgin of Fatima. It made me feel really good to know that she had spent some of her vacation time thinking about me and had gone to visit the place where the Virgin had appeared to children in order to pray for my recovery.

One day, I was taking Lilia's class about angels when I met a young Mexican girl that had recently married. When she heard of my problem, she brought me a bottle with holy oil from St. Charmain. She explained to me that this was a Lebanese saint to whom the Lebanese revered. She said this saint had helped her and her family in difficult moments and she asked me to put my life in his hands.

When Alejandro, who is one of my neighbors, found out about my condition, he talked to me about Sai Baba, a spiritual leader that he follows. He gave me a bag with some dust that he told me Sai Baba had materialized and given to him in person during one of his trips to India. Sai Baba had told him to share it with someone that had a real need for healing. He also has in his apartment one of Sai Baba's robes and he had invited me more than once to sit down in front of it and meditate, asking him for guidance and help.

One morning, I was visited by one of my neighbors from Ecuador. She had heard about my condition and wanted me to know that she and her family were praying for me. She brought me a small picture of the Virgin of the Holy Conception, to whom she and her family pray a lot. She then took me to her house to show me the beautiful altar that they had for her in her home, where she had put my picture so she could protect me.

One of the first gifts I received was from Antonio's mother, who sent me a silver figure of the Virgin of Rocío. They are very big followers of her and knew that she could protect me. Antonio's sister sent me a small gold medal with the likeness of the same virgin that I wore on my neck during some of my most difficult days.

From Mexico, my mother's sisters sent me a wide variety of rosaries from Mexico's patron, the Virgin of Guadalupe. Those rosaries were really special to me. I know they had to go through a lot to get them because they are very hard to find. I also know that they sent them with a lot of love and good intentions.

I could continue to mention the large number of religious or spiritual items that I received throughout my journey, but I don't think it is necessary. The important part of this story is not the material gift itself but what it meant to give and receive. Whoever was giving me something so special was showing me they had been thinking of me and were concerned about my situation. Every single one of those gifts represented love, faith, worries, and positive thoughts that people had toward me. Every time I received one of them, it was like a reaffirmation that my fight for life was worth it.

It is said faith can move mountains. Now that I have experienced this Difficult Journey, I have come to understand the meaning of this saying. Throughout this process of healing, I have seen that the faith you can have and the faith that others have can make it very possible for the healing to begin to happen.

During one of the days of my healing process, I had the opportunity to go to a luncheon in benefit of the American Cancer Society. I was able to acquire at their auction a beautiful silver cross, engraved with different religious symbols. I placed that cross on top of my bedroom dresser and I have hung on that cross all of the religious or spiritual gifts that I received during my illness. The place where that cross is has become my own little altar to thank the Supreme Being for all of the blessings I have received. During my illness, I was able to experience first hand the incredible power of praying, faith and positive thinking.

When they confirmed I had cancer, I was very surprised about the number of people who started calling me on the phone or contacting me by e-mail to give me their moral support and tell me that I was in their prayers. I'm not only talking about my close family and friends, but also about relatives with whom I did not have a close relationship, acquaintances I had only seen on a few occasions, and even people whom I hadn't had the chance to meet in person. I know they all prayed for me and my recovery. I was happily surprised to find out about the existence of some "prayer chains," through which people from different parts of the world, religions, cultures and beliefs get together every day at a certain time to pray for the healing of one particular person. It is truly admirable that there are some good people in the world who dedicate a good part of their day to pray for the well-being of others.

In this day of such advanced communications, it was very helpful to receive so many e-mails every single day. Although I wasn't physically able to reply to all of them, it boosted my self-esteem to know that so many people were concerned about my health on any given day. It's curious, but I've realized that e-mails often draw people together since we have a tendency to write what we really feel, which many times we are not able to express in the same manner on the phone or in person. A very special example of this for me was my cousin Eduardo. Even though we are first cousins, we never really talked much because he is a very introverted kind of guy. From the time he found out about my illness, he began writing to me constantly. I can honestly say his e-mails represented a ray of light that gave me strength and hope. He was always cheering me up and asking me not to give up. He kept sending me information about places where they were doing research on cancer. He became my link between my family in Mexico and me.

One of the most important issues during the recovery process is to be able to maintain a positive attitude so that we don't allow the illness to overcome us. Believe me, it's a lot easier said than done. I thought of giving up on some days during my process. Physically, I couldn't handle it anymore. Emotionally, I was very tired of fighting. Luckily for me, I always found that inner voice from the deepest part of my soul that kept pushing me and gave me the strength to face the situation.

We don't exactly know where cancer comes from. It's been proven that the cells begin to multiply in a disorderly fashion, creating what is called "cancer." There are many different kinds of cancer and multiple factors that influence its existence. In the case of breast cancer, there are various potentially decisive determinants that predispose a woman to have it: maternal heredity, having a first child after 35 years of age and high alcohol consumption. This kind of cancer is mostly present in women over 65 years of age. The younger a woman is when she has it, the more aggressive it tends to be. In my own family, neither my mother, grandmother nor sister had it. I gave birth to my two children before turning 31. I only drink alcohol socially. I was 38 on the day I found out I had cancer.

I have asked myself a thousand times why I have cancer if I do not fit its "medical profile." Now that I have had the opportunity of re-evaluating my life and analyzing my particular situation, I have discovered that the origin of my cancer is very specific. I have come to the conclusion that my cancer was the physical manifestation of a chain of bad feelings and energies that I had accumulated throughout the years. They were bad feelings that I hadn't liberated and emotional deceptions that I hadn't forgotten, as well as insecurities, sadness, loneliness, deceitfulness and feelings of rejection. Somehow, all these feelings and emotions were inside of me even though I thought I had let them go. Throughout the years, they stayed in my soul while I was disguising them, until one day they had to manifest themselves physically in my body. When adding to all of those bad feelings the tremendous amount of stress I had been dealing with for several years, my body had to react in some way. The reaction was cancer.

I honestly believe that, by not being able to channel all of those negative energies in a positive manner, the error manifested itself in the form of cancer. This is a very personal opinion formed after having lived through this experience and I do not expect everybody to be in agreement. From a scientific point of view, there is no way to prove the correlation between feelings and illnesses. From a spiritual point of view, the relationship does exist. Throughout my life I have been a person who tries to find the positive even within the negative. It reassures me to think that my illness manifested itself for this reason. This allows me the possibility of learning to release truly the negative feelings and to enjoy fully and completely the positive ones, from now on.

Just as I realized that many people have different beliefs, all of which are valid for each person, this is my belief and I choose to live with it.

CONCLUSION

My life hasn't been easy. My search hasn't been simple. This illness has given me the opportunity to reevaluate my life and look at it in a much more positive way. This illness has opened the eyes of my soul and taught me to change the order of my priorities. Not only have my priorities changed, but also the way I see, appreciate and enjoy life because I was very close to death. Your perspective of life changes when you see death from such a close proximity.

Healing has been a learning process and has made me a much more spiritual person. Now I am truly convinced that, in essence, we human beings are spirits and that our bodies are only an instrument lent to us to live while we are in the human condition. I finally understand that, when the time comes to leave, our body remains here on earth and disintegrates, but our soul rises and continues the journey. It is this conviction that makes me more courageous in the face of adversities. I am well aware that sooner or later we are all going to leave this earth. I know that the more obstacles I can conquer and the more tests I overcome, the more advanced spirit I will become. And the more advanced soul I become, the closer I will be to reaching eternal grace in the general plan of the universe.

I do not believe in coincidences. I believe that everything has a cause and effect. I know that everything in life happens for a reason. I am convinced that there is a very powerful reason for having lived A Difficult Journey that has taught me to become a better person. Besides helping me in my spiritual growth, it is helping a lot of those who have shared with me this difficult experience to be better people, rediscovering new facets of their souls that perhaps were dormant.

Maybe the only good thing to come out of this illness is the fact that, because I had to face it, I learned the meaning of true love. I was able to experience first hand unconditional love, pure love, spiritual love, sincere love and the love of friends. Besides all the love surrounding me during the whole process, I learned that there is a lot of compassion between human beings. Before this illness, I had heard about compassion, but I had never experienced it and would have never imagined that somebody could have this feeling toward me. Now that I have come across it first hand, I can say that compassion is a beautiful and pure quality that comes from the deepest part of the soul and generates wonderful energy.

One of the greatest lessons learned during the development of my problem was to feel and experience paternal love. Even though my father and I had grown apart from each other and I had grown up feeling his rejection, I finally felt his love toward me.

I have learned so very much during this year that if I had to return to this life to relive the experience, as painful and as difficult as it was, I would relive it. I have discovered the love of strangers. I have experienced kindness from people who, even in an oftentimes material society such as the one we live in, have lent helping hands. Although along the way I had a couple of unpleasant experiences, the overall situation has been good and positive.

This experience, as hard as it has been, has taught my children a lot. They also had to grow up, to face fear, to learn to be strong, and to support each other emotionally. They never stopped caring for me. They were always concerned about my health. They instinctively knew how to cheer me up even during the most difficult and dark days, making them easier to bear. Several times during my illness, especially during the beginning, I asked myself why two beautiful and innocent children had to be put through such a harsh lesson. I used to believe that childhood was supposed to be a happy period in life during which the major concern should be getting good grades in school and being good at home. Due to my illness, my children were forced to become much more responsible and stronger at a very young age. They were forced to confront doubt, anguish and fear—feelings that as a mother I would want to spare them from at all cost. Although we have been very fortunate and count on an excellent support team, I know that both of them suffered and were scared in their own way. I'm proud of them. They were always by my side. They learned to respect my need for time to be alone or to rest. They learned how to be brave. They learned how to cheer me up when I was sad or in pain. They made a huge effort to become the best students in their school, knowing it would make me very proud. They learned simple things such as bringing me a glass of water every morning as soon as I woke up. They also learned more responsible things such as giving me my medication at certain hours. My healing process was a team effort and my children played a very important role as an integral part of the team.

My friends, who as I said before became my spiritual family, also taught me very important lessons. With their friendship, support, time and dedication, they taught me the true meaning of friendship. The time that they shared with me visiting me, as well as taking me to the hospital, the doctor appointments or the treatments, was an invaluable help.

My sister and brothers showed me their support, each one in their own way. They all made me feel loved. Love enriches the soul.

The great majority of my doctors and the medical personnel that took care of me surrounded me with love, compassion and affection.

I am a very happy person and a more complete woman than I was a year and a half ago, when I didn't know that cancer was already inside my body. My values have changed and my quality of life has become better because I have come to know other aspects of people. Thanks to this illness, I am a better mother, daughter, friend and companion. I feel really happy having been capable of conquering this illness. I am eternally grateful to the universe and to my Lord, the Supreme Being, for giving me the opportunity to discover that this world is full of beautiful, noble and generous feelings.

Breast cancer is a very difficult illness, but it is an illness that bonds families and women of different races, religions, ages and social status, making us friends who identify with each other in the same fight: our race to reconquer life. We are women who live under the same uncertainty, pain and anguish. In the end, we are women who fight to defeat this illness because we have families that await us and some of us have children who need us, parents who miss us, and friends who support us.

Cancer is a difficult illness for the people who have it and for those who surround them. From the moment that we learn we have cancer, life hangs by a thread. Life changes drastically from night to day. Although we try hard to grab on to whatever we have in our quest to defeat it, it affects our relationships, families and jobs. In short, it changes our lives.

Despite being a cruel and treacherous illness, it is an illness that brings out the best feelings of those who surround us. In my particular case, the many blessings I found along the way and the goodness of people have made me a much better person.

I like to think that I never again will face something like what I have faced. I am not going to spend my life worrying about what might come tomorrow. Today I live my life fully each and every moment because I'm truly convinced that I am going to part this world only when my time is up and not a minute sooner nor a minute later. At the time of my departure, I want to be sure that I have lived a full life and that my soul is leaving filled with love and that I am much richer for all the spiritual wealth that I have accumulated along the way.

I love life. I am grateful to the universe for allowing me to experience A Difficult Journey. In one year of fighting to survive, I learned a lot more than in many years of joy.